AGING 2000

Disclaimers

The designations employed and the presentation of the material in this publication do not imply the expression of any opinion whatsoever on the part of the secretariat of the United Nations concerning the legal status of any country, territory, city, or area, or of its authorities, or concerning the delimitation of its frontiers or boundaries.

The editing and writing contributed to this book by Mal Schechter were in his private capacity. No official support or endorsement by the US National Institute on Aging, where he is an expert consultant, is intended or should be inferred.

AGING 2000
a challenge for society

Philip Selby   Mal Schechter

in collaboration with

Jean-Jacques Vollbrecht   Raymond Rigoni   Adrian Griffiths

in consultation with

United Nations Centre for Social Development and Humanitarian Affairs

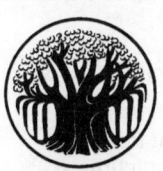

Published for

SANDOZ INSTITUTE FOR HEALTH AND SOCIO-ECONOMIC STUDIES

by

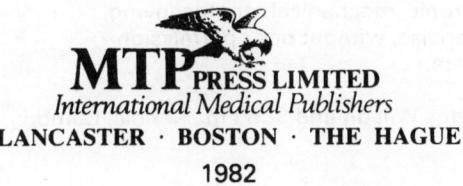

MTP PRESS LIMITED
International Medical Publishers
LANCASTER · BOSTON · THE HAGUE
1982

Published in the UK and Europe by
MTP Press Limited
Falcon House
Lancaster, England

British Library Cataloging in Publication Data

Aging 2000
  1. Aging
  I. Selby, P.   II. Schechter, M.

612'.67.   QP86

ISBN-13: 978-94-011-6275-3

Published in the USA by
MTP Press
A division of Kluwer Boston Inc
190 Old Derby Street
Hingham, MA 02043, USA

Library of Congress Cataloging in Publication Data

Selby, Philip, 1936-
Aging 2000: A Challenge for Society

Bibliography: P.
1. Aging.   2. Aging-Government Policy.
3. Social Surveys.   4. Social Prediction.
1. Schechter, Mal.   11. Title.

HQ1061.S43   1982   362.6   82-10110

ISBN-13: 978-94-011-6275-3   e-ISBN-13: 978-94-011-6273-9
DOI: 10.1007/ 978-94-011-6273-9

Typesetting by Titus Wilson and Son Ltd., Kendal, Cumbria

Cover by Peter Davies

Contents

Preface

> For age is opportunity no less
> Than youth itself, though in another dress,
> And as the evening twilight fades away
> The sky is filled with stars, invisible by day.
> Henry Wadsworth Longfellow, *Morituri Salutamus*

We live in a society that remorselessly casts off those who are too weak, mentally or physically, to cling to the dizzy wheel of existence – a society that worships the idols of beauty, youth, and wealth whilst ruthlessly rejecting those who fall outside its narrow standards of acceptability, or exploitability.

The elderly are the latest victims of an artificial life-style that tends to create artificial problems. In this respect, we have much to learn from those primitive communities that continue to revere their elders for the wisdom they have acquired in the school of life, and which have yet to make the dubious progression to a civilization that dismisses its senior members as senile old fools or a burden on taxpayers' funds. It is vital to warn developing countries of the dangers of duplicating the errors of the industrial world – of which they see only the superficial trappings that mask the iceberg of disillusionment beneath.

Many of the so-called problems of our time, of which the care of the elderly is just one example, are in fact manifestations of nature's resentment at man's unwarranted encroachment on her traditional territories. Rather than attempting to deal with these problems in isolation, usually by recourse to the very technology that helped cause them in the first place, it may prove more constructive to conduct an in-depth reappraisal of the philosophies that have caused humanity to take what is clearly a false turning.

One of the root causes of the rejection of the aged in our society is the breakdown of the fundamental contract of life, whereby care should be extended to the elderly as a right rather than as a privilege or, worse, a charity. It is the consideration to which the elderly are entitled, in return for a lifetime of devoted work and the care and

7

attention given to their children and grandchildren when they were dependent parties.

This agreement of honor, which continues largely to prevail in less developed countries, is disintegrating for several reasons. One is the gradual migration of populations towards large industrial complexes. The enforced crowding together of large communities in confined spaces has, ironically, signalled the erosion of the neighbor system — which in rural areas continues to watch over the well-being of the elderly, and to ensure that they are never totally divorced from the succour of society, even after the death of their spouses and relatives.

Another reason is the undue emphasis the industrialized world has placed on the concept of productivity, and on the remorseless disposal of assets, both human and material, once their usefulness has been exhausted.

It is a sad commentary on our times that telecommunications have brought the world into our living-rooms but have rendered us blind to the misery next door! This situation must not be allowed to become self-perpetuating. A more constructive, crisis-management approach is called for — less piecemeal and sectorial — in developing integrated action programs to counter the problems of modern living.

At the same time, we must take steps to instill in our youth a new sensitivity which will allow them to temper their fascination for leisure, sensuality, and materialism with renewed awareness of the counsel of the wise, and a return to understanding and respect for age. Most importantly, future generations must not be encouraged, directly or indirectly, by the authorities, the media, the technocrats — or indeed by the present report — to look upon their elders as potential problems or burdens. Rather, the provision of prosperity, health, and happiness for senior citizens must be based on sincere sentiments of esteem, comprehension, compassion, and tolerance — to which the donors will in turn be entitled in the autumn of their lives. The accent must be on need, rather than on age.

Another fundamental reason for the apparent failure of our society to come to terms with old age is that, whilst the advance of science has helped to push back the frontiers of longevity, our civilization has removed much of the will to live that would render the exercise worthwhile. Symptomatically, we have endeavored to hold mortality in check by recourse to chemical crutches that support the elderly through the years they have cheated from nature. This approach has, in many ways, proved counter-productive. Notably, it has given rise to a cultural myth that, directly one has attained a certain age, one is automatically a deserving case for medical treatment.

Upon closer examination, the elixir of youth would seem to flow, not so much from the fountain of science, as from a sense of self-preservation, born out of a feeling that there is something left to achieve – something worth living for.

History supplies abundant examples of late-life accomplishment, which refute the popular presumption that success and fulfilment must necessarily diminish with advancing years. Indeed, countless scientists, writers, and artists have continued to make significant contributions (and even produce their masterpieces) late in life. (Whether the same is true of politicians and statesmen remains a matter of some controversy!)

Thus, it would seem that much could be achieved by restoring to the individuals who make up our society – and especially to our youth, the elderly of tomorrow – a sense of identity and purpose, together with a renewed awareness of their true position in the cosmic cycle of all things. Old age, like death, is a natural process – part of life itself – that should be prepared for in an atmosphere of serenity. It is not an ominous specter, which deserves to be hidden from society or banished to specialized institutions.

Rather than being needlessly stigmatized or segregated, there are many areas in which the elderly may continue to play useful roles in society following retirement. Such activity constitutes a source of motivation which, together with regular exercise, sensible diet, the cultivation of an active mind, and spiritual fulfilment, may prove of greater long-term value than the plethora of tranquilizers, anti-depressants, and cerebral vasodilators that are sold each year. We must learn to treat the civilization and life-style that continue to incubate the malaise, rather than merely the symptoms.

Human problems – which vary so greatly between individuals – do not easily lend themselves to general solutions that will prove satisfactory in all cases. This is especially true in an international context, when dealing with people and communities of vastly different backgrounds, aspirations, and creeds. The greatest danger clearly lies in attempting to impose – by means of international conventions – solutions conceived to meet one set of circumstances, which later prove to be hopelessly ill-adapted or totally inadequate when transposed to a different cultural or social environment.

In this context, the greatest sufferers are, too often, the inhabitants of less developed countries. They tend to inherit inappropriate, western-designed solutions and shortly afterwards – by a curious back-to-front process – the problems to match! Our western society created the problem of the elderly, which it has attempted to solve, largely unsuccessfully, by recourse to institutions. Let us not encourage developing countries to build institutions and then seek out the elderly to fill them!

We must cast aside our paternalistic attitude and blind belief in the superiority of the industrialized system. Let us take a more humble approach. Before indulging in wholesale westernization, let us investigate whether we have something to learn – or more likely re-discover – from the traditions that prevail in Third-World nations.

Relationships with developing countries should never be looked upon as a one-way traffic in ideas. They may teach us much about the quality of life, and even – judging from the life-spans of certain peoples in the Caucasus or the Andes – about the secret of longevity.

Another criticism, often levelled against those responsible for the implementation of international action programs, is the distressing tendency to consider that a problem may be solved merely by being defined. This results in interminable lapses into what Harold Laski termed "that state of resentful coma which at universities is called research". The temptation is to postpone the moment of confrontation, by circumventing the issues and cataloguing them in abstract study papers and statistics that will forever gather dust on library shelves.

Hopefully, this danger may be averted, with respect to the World Assembly on Aging, if the delegates constantly bear in mind that they are likely to be among the first beneficiaries, or victims, of the reforms they hope to implement. We are dealing with people, not statistics. Aging is something that most of us will be confronted with sooner or later. Therefore we are likely to derive a more humane, less technical or theoretical approach to this most natural of processes if we each devote some thought to how we ourselves would wish to be treated in the autumn of our lives.

Certainly, judging from the rich treasure-chest of varied data – covering all aspects of the aging process – assembled in the present study, we cannot complain of any lack of authoritative documentation to facilitate our task. But no change can come from a bureaucratic approach, however competent the experts. It must come from the heart. Will this report spark the awareness that can contribute to such a change?

Let us hope that the investment in a World Assembly on Aging will be more than justified in terms of lasting benefit for the elderly, both of this generation and of those to come.

Sadruddin Aga Khan,
Geneva

Introduction

This book reports the findings of an international survey on the problems of the elderly, carried out by the Sandoz Institute in consultation with the United Nations Centre for Social Development and Humanitarian Affairs. It is offered both as a contribution to the World Assembly on Aging (Vienna, 26 July to 6 August 1982) and as a text for study and discussion in government, academic, community, religious, philanthropic, trade-union, and corporate organizations. For the purpose of the survey, and to conform with official usage for the Assembly, the elderly were defined as persons aged 60 and over.

Many nations find themselves with larger populations of elderly persons than ever before. Demographic aging is a consequence of falling birth rates and increasing life expectancy, themselves a reflection of improved living standards and health care. As the title of this volume states, the world is faced with a challenge. This must not be construed only as a challenge to meet problems – it is also a challenge to recognize and make use of new potentials. In the more developed countries, the problems for society and for elderly individuals themselves are already felt acutely. In many countries at an earlier stage of development, the problems are barely perceived directly, are beginning to be understood vicariously, and thus are recognized as likely to become severe unless suitable and timely measures are taken.

Our survey aimed to identify these problems in sixteen countries at various levels of development and in all regions of the world, and to foresee how they might evolve up to the end of this century. It also set out to explore what measures exist in these countries for dealing with their problems. In this way, it sought to help nations to learn from one another. Finally, it attempted to stimulate ideas for future action which might help to guide policy-makers.

The participating countries were: Australia, Brazil, Egypt, Federal Republic of Germany, France, India, Israel, Italy, Japan, Kenya, Nigeria, Philippines, Poland, Sweden, UK, and USA. Questionnaire responses were provided in each country by a small working group of three experts, representing the broad areas of health, sociology,

11

and social policy, often with additional advisors. In Israel, a consensus response was obtained from a large number of experts at one institute of gerontology, as well as outside advisors.

The first round of the survey was based on 17 topics: maintaining an active and independent life for as long as possible, preventing and coping with chronic physical and mental disorders, ensuring suitable housing, enabling the elderly to remain in their own homes for as long as possible, provision of institutional services, provision of community-based and home services, payment for health and social services, optimal utilization of human resources, support by the family, role in the family, support by the community, role in the community, activities and the use of time, ensuring an adequate income after retirement, employment policies, preparation for retirement, and retirement policies. For each topic the same four questions were posed:

- What are the main problems today?
- What policies and programs exist for dealing with them?
- What main problems do you foresee in the year 2000?
- What measures, including novel and unconventional ones, should in your opinion be undertaken in order to reduce or prevent these problems?

In addition, the experts were asked to rank a list of nine subjects, covered by the first round of the survey, in their order of importance in their own country – "important" in the sense that problems exist for which measures are urgently needed. The subjects are: health, housing, health services and social services, family, community, activities, income, work and employment, and retirement. The responses are presented graphically in the relevant sections.

A second round dealt with a few important issues on which it was felt that further elaboration would be useful: the diversity of the elderly, employment, research, and political factors in policy-making.

In the course of the survey the importance of economic factors became increasingly apparent. We therefore invited a distinguished expert, Brian Abel-Smith, to contribute an Economic Commentary.

This volume is the culmination of a group endeavor by many people. Through their efforts we hope we have succeeded in producing a report which will interest and stimulate a wide international readership among people of diverse backgrounds and interests. As the survey was begun in November 1980 we were faced throughout by a crucial time constraint. Only the devoted efforts of all who took part enabled us to carry it out, analyze the responses, and prepare and publish the report in time for the World Assembly on Aging.

INTRODUCTION

Our sincere thanks are due to the many distinguished experts who participated in our survey, and whose names are listed in the report. We also wish to acknowledge the valuable support provided by Sandoz Ltd. in 13 of the countries, where they undertook the task of selecting and inviting the experts, organizing and reporting the working group discussions, and liaising with the Sandoz Institute. Without this logistic support such a broad international survey would have been impossible within the limited time available. In the three other countries (Israel, Nigeria, and Poland) the role of coordinator was kindly performed by Michael Davies, Olatunji Adeniyi-Jones, and Zbigniew Brzezinski, respectively.

The report has benefited by additional contributions. We are greatly indebted to Sadruddin Aga Khan for his Preface, and to Leo Kaprio and Eyvind Hytten, of WHO and the UN, respectively, for their comments.

We are especially indebted to Mal Schechter for his thorough analysis of the experts' replies, his valuable suggestions in preparing the second round of the survey, and his major role in drafting the final report.

The survey was conceived, planned, and carried out by the Sandoz Institute research team. Philip Selby, who directed the project, was mainly responsible for its methodological aspects and for editing the final report, of which he is co-author. Jean-Jacques Vollbrecht dealt with much of the planning and administration, particularly coordination with the experts and with Sandoz Ltd. in the various participating countries. Adrian Griffiths and I participated in developing the methodology and advised on the drafting of the report. Christine Emamzadah dealt efficiently with the large amount of secretarial work involved. This teamwork was an essential component of the whole endeavor.

We hope this survey will help to draw the attention of policy-makers, and all who are concerned about the aging of societies, to some of the pressing needs in this vast area. The report suggests that most countries have not found adequate solutions to the problems caused by the aging of their populations, indeed many do not even have the beginning of adequate social policies for preventing or coping with such problems. There appears to be an urgent need for more information about the elderly and aging societies, as a basis for sound policies and programs.

If this report helps to stimulate further research and action, the efforts of its many contributors will have been amply rewarded.

Raymond Rigoni, director,
Sandoz Institute for health and socio-economic studies

Overall summary

Policy-making for the later years of life has paused at a perceived but unexplored frontier in many countries around the world.

The growth of elderly populations is unmistakable. But the profound implications for today and tomorrow are only dimly perceived by policy-makers.

Demographic and other trends have undermined many public and private policies and programs, and their underlying attitudes and philosophies concerning working life and retirement, pension finance, provision of health and social services, living arrangements, and contributions that older people can make to their societies and themselves.

Issues may have been raised but practical solutions have not been thought through in many countries, perhaps most notably on two major concerns. One is long-term care, typically poorly organized and financed. Secondly, an enormous policy void exists on jobs for the elderly — chiefly the specific issues of delaying retirement and creating opportunities for productive and satisfying activities after retirement. Policies and programs for well and sick elders often are conceived, inaugurated, and maintained on a token or fragmented basis. To do otherwise may conflict with well-established priorities in allocation of social resources: for example, the young want jobs held by the elderly; health-care providers do not want to disturb economic arrangements favoring acute over long-term care.

Looming over the major issues is ageism, or deeply rooted discrimination against the elderly.

In many countries, no coherent approach is evident to resolving many fundamental problems by the year 2000. By and large, problems seen today will worsen for the elderly. Notably, trends towards earlier retirement are seen intensifying in many countries, and income-maintenance programs will be hard pressed to provide for more years in retirement.

The foregoing statements represent a consensus of experts on aging, in 16 countries, who responded to a survey by the Sandoz Institute on problems of the elderly. The experts reviewed problems

15

within contemporary contexts and with an eye to the coming two decades.

Many nations are experiencing inflation, especially in health-care services (relied on heavily by the elderly). Many also are experiencing economic stagnation and recession, which erode their abilities, through social insurance and other programs, to provide for the elderly.

And there are varying trends in fertility. In some developed nations, the ratio of elderly to working-age population is increasing, though the ratio of child dependents to elderly population appears to be declining. In less developed nations, the youth component of total dependency ratio is far higher than the elder component, and is likely to remain so.

The World Assembly on Aging comes at a propitious time. Problems are being defined. New approaches to problems are being discussed or attempted. Governments increasingly are in a mood to learn from one another about programs and policies. Moreover, a sense of urgency is developing in recognition of the relatively long intervals needed to prepare and accomplish institutional reforms, and the relatively short intervals before the larger populations arrive at old age, particularly the post-World War II "baby boomers" in some of the more developed countries.

High birth rates and reduced death rates are enlarging the populations of the less developed countries at a rapid rate, setting the stage for their future elderly populations. Preparations not made within the next few years may be impossible or difficult to make, and to synchronize with the arrival of larger cohorts of elderly persons.

Policy is difficult to frame when the diversity of the elderly population is poorly comprehended. The population called "elderly", from age 60 or 65, spans three decades or more. The diversity of this population is sensed, but unevenly appreciated, by the public at large and even by the elderly themselves.

It includes many healthy, vigorous individuals who are able and willing to work or to participate actively in leisure, family, and civic affairs. Many can lead active lives with some assistance. Many are dependent on housing, health, social, and other services to continue living at home. And some are so dependent on others that they must have the kind of continuous and expert attention available only in a hospital or skilled nursing home.

An individual may have a progressive course of decline through these stages of dependency before dying. The experts generally see that support systems are incomplete or uncoordinated and that the elderly themselves often cannot afford the services they need, if the services are at all available or within reach at any price.

An individual may require relatively little supportive service to remain active in a desired style of life, provided there are opportunities for self-expression and self-support through paid employment, volunteer work, and recreational or cultural activities. Retirement for vigorous elderly people may be a personal disaster under circumstances of poverty, inadequate preparation for using free time, prejudice against the elderly, loneliness, boredom, and poor housing and transportation.

Thus, the population and its needs establish a policy-making frontier of enormous size and complexity. It is all the more complicated by general inflation and economic problems.

Identifying the needs but often no serious processes for dealing with them, the experts look at the future pessimistically, whether they are in developed countries, such as the United States and in Western Europe, or in less developed countries, such as India and Nigeria. One would be hard put to find a more pessimistic statement than one from an Australian expert. After surveying inflation, the difficulties of increasing employment, and other conditions, the expert comments:

". . . without wishing to sound too much of a Jeremiah, I believe that there are no solutions in sight for our socio-economic decline, and that the old haven't got a chance."

In Sweden, a nation with highly advanced programs for the elderly, there is concern whether today's standards of living and service for the elderly can be maintained. In other countries, the experts fear that needed progress to a decent level will not occur. In Brazil, where problems of general unemployment are deeply rooted, the experts see no hope that the elderly will receive financial support. While many experts see that an expanding economic base is needed for funding solutions for the elderly, they do not foresee an adequate pace.

In the shadow of pessimism deriving from the immensity of needs and the paucity of clear policy directions and commitments, one may find occasional optimism. After all, the experts note, the needs result from an astonishing improvement in average life expectancy in the past 150 years in the industrial nations, and in a shorter span for less developed countries. If there is a basis for pessimism about the future, there also is a basis for optimism: the forces that produced longer life and vigor can be harnessed to reduce or eliminate the problems that have accompanied them. Retrospectively, one can say that many of the directions taken by societies were not clearly foreseen 50 or even 20 years ago. The problems so conspicuous today may not endure, while less obtrusive problems may come to the fore.

Nonetheless, there is a cost to be paid in ignoring the problems and leaving matters entirely to chance, or to forces that provide for old age as a by-product of their principal thrusts. The cost of ignoring problems may be measured partly as costs to society of large populations that are kept relatively unproductive for longer and longer intervals. These are costs in earnings foregone, in the depressive personal, familial, and community consequences of frustrated and deprived lives, and in broader national consequences of medical and social care expenses.

It is measured, too, in the message given tacitly to young as well as old: after working life, the individual is not of much self or societal value.

It may well be that one source of prejudice against the elderly population – a prejudice that is reported in all the countries, with possible exceptional enclaves in non-industrialized areas – is fear among the young of joining the ranks of the ignored and disposable. This may be a hidden morale problem around the world. The magnitude in any country may parallel its degree of urbanization and industrialization, that is, its distance from agrarian, family-centered traditions.

The experts also point out that tomorrow's elderly – today's middle-aged – may be quite different in outlook from today's elderly. Their social history, as well as their economic status, will surely be different. Today's elderly populations generally lack the group consciousness necessary for political organization and activity. However, it is conceivable that tomorrow's elderly may, in some degree, engage in age-based politics. This is seen by some experts as being more likely where governments and political parties fail to respond seriously to problems produced by age prejudice.

Lacking at the policy-making frontier, the experts suggest, is the concept that attending to the problems of the elderly is synonymous with attending to the problems confronting those who are now young. Indeed, the life cycle should be addressed in many nations as a fundamental planning concept. Problems and potentials in later life are prepared for in early life. Difficulties facing the elderly today may be experienced later by those who are now middle-aged.

The experts are concerned about inter-generational conflicts but tend to feel that, if these are real, they represent conflicts between the needs an individual experiences in earlier life and those that he or she will experience later on. This is very much like the conflict between spending now and saving for later. To the extent that problems of old age are not perceived as potentially one's own problems, major cues for political action and social planning will be missing. This consciousness, however, may be growing as today's younger adults confront their roles in assisting their parents and grandparents in coping with longer lives.

Thus, the experts would place their pessimism in context: matters will tend to worsen for the elderly unless new perspectives about them, and the challenges and opportunities for policy-making, are examined and acted upon.

What are the main theaters for action? With some variation arising partly from whether the expert was in a more developed or less developed nation, here are the major themes:

1. Jobs and the able-bodied elderly

As standards of living rise, including preservation of health and vigor later and later in the lifespan, national economies appear to have little if any room for able-bodied men and women who want to continue working into and beyond their 60s. Dependency on government and private pension programs is fostered. These programs, however, are seen as verging on bankruptcy or as causing severe burdens on the population of conventional working age, perhaps intensifying their hostility toward the elderly. This is the "taxpayers' revolt".

If, indeed, a shortage of jobs exists or will worsen, should the exclusion of the elderly be accepted?

If jobs will be in short supply, how should they be allocated – at random, by special interests acting on their own, or by some reasoned public policy?

Will societies desire to invent ways of sharing jobs throughout the life cycle, if they are not able or willing to create enough jobs for all?

While the experts generally see a need for extending the conventional span of working life, they are uncertain about national capacities to do so in the light of inflationary and other economic trends.

The experts worry not only about the economic security of older persons, but also about their mental health when deprived of a central pivot of their lives. People who have organized their lives around the material and psychic benefits of paid employment may well be unprepared for leisure, and may not want it. Those needing more money than their pensions provide are particularly disadvantaged because of work limitations attached to pensions and the stigma attached to poverty.

2. The ill elderly and services

Turning from the able-bodied to the elderly in compromised health, the experts see a population for which housing, health, and social arrangements are generally deficient. In most of the countries covered by the Sandoz Institute survey, the population needing these arrangements – more likely to be those over age 75 or 80 than younger – is growing at a faster pace than almost any other age group.

Again and again, the experts characterize problems for this group as worsening by the year 2000. These include shortages of (a) geriatrically oriented or trained professionals in medicine, nursing, and social services and less-trained individuals who serve as home helps and other attendants; (b) nursing homes, day-care centers, and home-health agencies; (c) housing, and support services designed for tenants of congregate housing who need assistance in caring for themselves; (d) effective procedures of diagnosis, treatment, or prevention related to processes of aging and chronic disease.

3. The elderly and families

Break-up of the larger family – due to urbanization and industrialization – emerges as a major problem for both the well and sick elderly. In both more developed and less developed nations, pressure on younger family members to migrate for job purposes means two things to the elders: they may be left behind because they do not want to leave familiar surroundings; they may accept crowding and new, possibly demeaning, roles when they move with their adult children.

Whatever the reason for separation, it means that elderly couples or persons lose actual or potential assistance from their grown children. They may also lose usual family and community roles. If they move in with working children, a major change in health status – particularly a need for continued or chronic care during the working day – may become a source of tension within the family. It may force the children to seek institutional care for the elders.

As women tend more and more to find careers outside the household, sickness in an elderly member becomes less and less manageable in the family. Yet despite serious internal frictions, families stay in contact. Younger members often make sacrifices, up to a point, to prevent institutionalization.

The experts note that society has a major stake in the ability of families to care for their elders. Of all social institutions, the family is the source of the overwhelming bulk of support given to the elderly population. When the family is no longer willing or able to provide support, the needs of the elderly may be unmet or may be answered in some measure by community, philanthropic, religious, and governmental organizations. The longer families can be supported and encouraged to care for their elders, the less may be the need or demand for services by formal organizations. These formal services tend to be more expensive and less satisfying than the family assistance they would replace. They might be far more costly than direct payments to families and other forms of family cash or service support; the experts generally would like to see this point researched as an aid to policy-makers.

Further, the experts are concerned about specific policies to support the principal care-givers within the family, who may need counseling, training, and professional services in order to accept and be effective with the elders.

Few if any policies aimed at aiding families through subsidies, special at-home or outpatient services, transportation, and housing arrangements are found by the experts. Few countries have comprehensive programs that allow a diversity of options for a diversity of circumstances. Housing policy, for example, rarely supports constructing or renovating apartment buildings in order to offer meals and health, social, and other services. Such services can be brought into play during episodes of poor health or as dependency progressively increases. Indeed, the experts observe that some domiciliary programs produce better health, principally through improved social support.

Few countries provide for construction or renovation of space in family-owned property for "granny annexes". There are only rare programs to subsidize the rents of the poor elderly and to help them maintain or adapt their housing so it is clean, safe, and free of barriers to movement.

The absence of flexible programs can be seen as a risk to survival of body and of personal identity. For example, when family aid is exhausted, there is little else for the elderly person in many countries than admission to a nursing home or hospital that will serve the poor. By and large, the elderly who outrun family aid already have exhausted their own financial resources, or soon will become impoverished. Bereft of family and income support, the elderly person is at risk of physical and mental breakdown; in many countries, high suicide rates are noted in the elderly population. Because of deficiencies in the health and social care system, admission to an institution is the only feasible course of action. It often may exacerbate depression, produce boredom, and increase feelings of insignificance and abandonment.

Nor do the experts generally find adequate systems of services, and adequate personnel, to help maintain the elderly person in his or

21

her community. Some reluctance to provide even the less-skilled services of housekeepers and chore persons is found in some countries. There is fear that such steps would encourage families to do less, and thereby shift costs prematurely to the public sector and more expensive providers of care.

The issue may be open to research and demonstration, as are others. The experts are left to wonder, along with policy-makers, what, indeed, would be the effects on the family and institutional placements if a variety of resources were available at home or on an outpatient basis, such as:

– respite care (permitting the family to vacation while a disabled elder is supervised in a health-care or congregate-living facility);

– day care (providing supervision, rehabilitation, recreational therapy, meals, and other services while family members are away from home during the work day);

– home care (by means of visiting nurses and therapists, home helps, and delivered meals);

– various housing and transportation arrangements.

4. The elderly and the life cycle

Preparation for a long life involves societal and personal actions throughout the life cycle. Putting aside genetic issues, the experts would like policy-makers to consider that the biomedical, psychological, and socio-economic condition of the individual in old age reflects his or her past. Many problems of old age require solutions that begin in earlier life. For example, saving and participation in pension and social-security systems; adoption of good nutritional and exercise patterns; obtaining guidance on, and practicing, a healthy life style (including habits of dealing with emotional stress); arrangements for medical care (including preventive medicine and self-care practice); development of recreational and other leisure interests. The reduction of morbidity and mortality rates through general programs of public health – including sanitation, immunization, and nutrition – has been largely responsible for longer lives in both more developed and less developed countries.

Many experts express particular concern about retirees' ability to handle their leisure time and to find post-employment roles which they, and society at large, will accept and support as worthwhile. The experts see desirable roles for older persons in the community and the family. They offer suggestions that range from a public service corps uniting older and younger persons, to a kind of foster grand-parenting. A role is advanced for the elderly in rearing the younger members of families whose parents are busy in their work careers.

Preparation for retirement, usually reserved for the immediately preceding years, probably should begin in youth. Some experts suggest that schools should convey the concept of developing the whole person, not primarily those functions related to earning a living. Adult education is seen as a lifelong activity, with rewards in continual mental refreshment. Universities of the Third Age, an innovation in adult education, are mentioned as one type of institution deserving further development.

Some experts believe that affordable, accessible health-care services throughout life are essential to a satisfying old age; particularly noted is the value of anti-hypertension screening and therapy, in preventing stroke and other cardiovascular diseases common in old age. This viewpoint suggests that programs for the elderly are, indeed, programs for the young. In this sense, inter-generational conflicts over resources have a basis for being harmonized. They may be seen as conflicts in priorities rather than conflicts over ultimate goals.

5. The elders as resources

Modern societies appear to ignore the skills and abilities of a large fraction of their populations: the elderly. In both less developed and more developed nations, prejudice against older people – sometimes when they are no older than 35 – produces or confirms their continued unemployment.

The experts see much of their countries' elderly populations as having positive contributions to make (a) to society at large, through volunteer and family roles, through small businesses created by or for the elderly, and through advisory or part-time jobs; (b) to their communities; and (c) to organizations which serve other elderly persons. Some experts urge that the elderly participate in making organizational decisions and in carrying them out. The elders can be mutually supportive, if they have the mechanisms and encouragement to perform in this way.

Emphasis on the "burdens" of the elderly population often reflects a dearth of imagination in the public and private sectors. Because forecasts of growth of national economies influence discussions about providing for later life, the Sandoz Institute requested an economic commentary to supplement the views of the experts in gerontology (see p. 177).

To be sure, planning for the elderly does not occur in a vacuum. "The wealth out of which to provide for the sick and disabled, and to provide for years of retirement or dependency, cannot be created fast enough unless human resources are fully usable," says Dr Halfdan Mahler, director-general of the World Health Organization.

Those resources surely include the elderly themselves.

CORE ISSUE FROM ROUND ONE

(replies by country)

MAINTAINING AN ACTIVE AND INDEPENDENT LIFE FOR AS LONG AS POSSIBLE

The UN, in its call for the World Assembly, uses the phrase: "Older people as contributors to and not just the beneficiaries of development". This is not just an ideal hope, if we believe that many older people are demonstrably competent and that more could be if we worked at it.

This kind of optimism does not discount a minority of older persons with extensive functional impairment under the best of circumstances. But the size of this minority matters, and is potentially modifiable. This potential modifiability is *the* subject of public policy for aging societies.

George Maddox
Duke University, Durham, N.C.

Maintaining an active and independent life for as long as possible

AUSTRALIA

The main problems today

Most aged cope well in society. For a minority, yet to be quantified, the main problems are:

– Lack of a purpose and joy in life.

– Lack of a positive image for old age: few acknowledged vocational or "voluntary" roles; limited access to meaningful social roles; decreased family role and relationships.

– Social isolation, from other individuals and from the community.

– Chronic physical and/or mental disability and a feeling that decay and disability are inevitable.

– Adverse socio-economic factors, such as inadequate income and poor housing.

Policies and programs today

Apart from a sustained campaign against smoking, and a lot of advice on diet, little has been done in the field of health promotion, health education, self-care, and preventive geriatrics. However, the National Heart Foundation has promoted regular blood pressure and other checks, and increasing numbers of people in and over middle age are having their hypertension and other cardiovascular problems treated.

Ordinary medical care is readily available within the means of most elderly people, through arrangements made for pensioners and the disadvantaged, or through general health-insurance arrangements for others. Care is available free of charge at recognized public hospitals, but only a limited number have specialist geriatric services.

Voluntary, especially religious, organizations provide home help and residential services to the elderly.

Government financial support is provided for "senior citizens' centers", which cater to the recreational needs of people aged 55 and older. Concessions are available to age pensioners for driving licence fees; theater, cinema, and sports complex charges; holiday rail travel; holiday tours; and entry to national parks.

Continuing education is obtainable, usually at a cost.

The year 2000

Little change is expected from 1980. Socio-economic factors will be increasingly adverse because of the relatively large growth in numbers of the elderly. For the same reason, there will be proportionately more disability in the population. The elderly will have an even less clear-cut role in, and possibly support from, the family, hence even greater isolation.

There is likely to be overwhelming pressure on families to care for frail, confused parents, because of inadequacy of a suitable, diversified system of care, including a balance between permanent institutional care and community-based services. As a consequence, a return to more custodial ("warehouse") institutions is likely. A high rate of breakdown in family support systems is likely, in the face of increased stress.

Most chronic diseases will come under greater control. However, psycho-geriatric problems will still be taking their toll.

Recommendations

1. Promote flexible retirement policies.

2. Educate the public to accept roles outside of conventional work, such as participation in organizations like the Retired Senior Volunteer Program.

3. Improve education and training in geriatrics at undergraduate and postgraduate levels, for all relevant categories of health personnel.

4. Educate for aging in schools, community, and mass media.

5. Establish "area" geriatric units covering not more than 200,000 people each, with these functions:

- health promotion and health education of direct relevance to maintaining an active and independent life;
- screening of persons at risk and arrangement of necessary services;
- assessment, treatment, and rehabilitation of disabled persons on referral;

— advice to government, voluntary organizations, and private practitioners.

6. Establish an "Aged award" system, similar to the Duke of Edinburgh award and Outward Bound courses for youth. (The Duke of Edinburgh award scheme offers young people, aged 14 to 25, challenging opportunities to participate in a wide range of practical, adventurous, community, and physical activities. The Outward Bound courses place each participant in an environment (such as a wilderness) to face challenges, make new discoveries about himself or herself, and build self-reliance, self-confidence, and social understanding.)

BRAZIL

The main problems today

Owing to a low level of education, including health education, people generally are unaware of the necessity for improving their own health. Preventive geriatrics is not practiced, owing perhaps to a lack of information and professional training. Arteriosclerosis is responsible for much disability and death in later life. Nutrition is poor. Low income does not allow for a reasonably healthy life.

Because of long commuting times, workers in urban areas have no opportunity to develop leisure activities.

Policies and programs today

Policies and programs directed at the foregoing problems are weak, but about the best the country can afford because of scanty resources.

The year 2000

Social services will be even more overtaxed as the number of elderly persons rises. Serious mental health problems will occur.

Recommendations

1. Combat age prejudice and discrimination by various means, including the schools.

2. Orient government and the private sector to regard all efforts to improve later life as medium-term investments in human capital.

3. Give the working population training and encouragement to engage in recreational activities.

EGYPT

The main problems today

Because there is little recognition of the needs of the elderly, there is little response to them. Among these needs are: greater involvement in community life; part-time jobs after retirement; activity programs and rehabilitation; specialized medical care, especially physiotherapy and mental health care; and preventive geriatrics. Family members and neighbors have particular needs for information about the physiological changes and diseases prevalent in old age. Medication dosages are not adjusted to take account of age changes. Insufficient attention is given to nutrition of the elderly.

Most Egyptians lack education in good physical and mental health practices, including regular physical exercise, sports, hobbies, and other leisure activities.

Policies and programs today

Geriatric research, training, and care programs are rare: the geriatric research center in Alexandria University, started in 1965, has 20 beds and a weekly outpatient service. A course in geriatrics is given for undergraduate medical students, and there are lectures for postgraduates.

Health insurance theoretically covers retirees upon payment of 1% of their monthly pension, and widows of retirees upon payment of 2%. However, the coverages are being phased in, as circumstances permit.

Five clubs for the elderly – or day-care centers – have been established experimentally as an American-Egyptian project in four cities. The centers offer activity programs, vocational training, recreation, and trips.

Little is being done to increase public awareness. A TV program directed mainly to the elderly helps to some extent. A society for senior citizens has been formed by the ministry of social affairs, which also conducts training sessions for social workers in which needs of the elderly are covered.

The year 2000

Diseases related to modern life will increase. With more urbanization and industrialization, alienation and health problems will increase. Because of rising life expectancy and a larger elderly population, more services will be needed but resources will be lacking. More burdens will fall on the family, unless institutions are created to help.

The economic prospects do not favor the elderly: jobs and occupational training for the elderly will not be available; economic pressures may force the government to remove the subsidies for medications and special foods; despite government efforts, pension raises will not keep up with inflation.

Recommendations

1. Promote preventive geriatrics and an inter-disciplinary approach to services, including medical, social, psychological, and other disciplines.

2. Establish more day-care centers, clubs, homes for the aged, and other residential facilities for the elderly.

3. Cover all the needy elderly with health insurance.

4. Promote programs of health education, to prepare the middle-aged for old age and to educate families about the needs of the elderly.

5. Increase research to determine safe and effective drugs and dosages for the elderly with specific ailments.

6. Establish a Supreme Council for the Elderly, to help make policies and coordinate programs.

7. Make occupational therapy, vocational training, and part-time jobs available for the elderly.

FEDERAL REPUBLIC OF GERMANY

The main problems today

Impediments to an active life in old age originate mostly in youth and middle age. They begin with poor health education in youth.

Middle age is marked by a sedentary lifestyle; too little cultivation of social contacts; nutritional defects; little interest (in certain population groups) in providing for old age; lack of leisure interests and hobbies; and professional over-work, especially by older employees. An active life in old age is impeded by the lack of a supportive-services system for people with minor handicaps; a lack of consider-

31

ation for the specific needs of the elderly in the equipment of dwellings, in the devices used in everyday life, and in transportation; and difficulty in keeping up with technological changes.

Doctors show little interest in patient education. The elderly lack practical information on health maintenance. Rehabilitation measures are insufficiently studied. Information through the mass media often causes anxiety or builds false hopes. Numerous programs may miss their targets; for example, leisure activities programs are often used by those who need them least.

Policies and programs today

The following programs exist but are scarce, unevenly distributed and staffed, and inadequately coordinated: home-delivered social and other services, outpatient services, day clinics, senior centers, adult education, group gymnastics, rehabilitation services, information and referral services.

The year 2000

Many problems will diminish (especially in the health area) owing to successful income-maintenance measures, a heightened consciousness of health, and medical progress (for example, further development of orthopedic prostheses and heart operations). But the increase in the number of the very old will be accompanied by an increase in the amount of physical handicap and mental illness.

Because of improved education, older people will develop leisure interests and participate in social and civic activities. A reduction in working hours will yield increased free time starting in middle age, and result in more physical exercise.

Recommendations

1. Promote sensible nutritional and living habits.

2. Improve health education.

3. Train doctors in geriatrics and gerontology.

4. Establish special services to aid the elderly.

5. Encourage the middle-aged to participate in non-competitive sports.

FRANCE

The main problems today

1. Lack of services, income, and other supports for the dependent elderly.

2. Denial of self-support opportunities for the independent or autonomous elderly.

3. The failure of society to provide – and of the elderly to adopt – civic, family, and personal development activities that make constructive and satisfying use of the time of retirees.

Meeting the needs of a growing elderly population surely requires broad social planning, not piecemeal or stop-gap programming for the elderly alone.

There are several key aspects to maintaining an independent life. One is to have assistance in minimizing dependency and disability. Another is financial sufficiency, including opportunity for paid employment. For those who are well-off financially and have their health as well as for those who are dependent, there must be preparation for an active, satisfying life in retirement. The retired person should be encouraged to participate in community life (especially in civic service), in family life (including helping to educate grandchildren), and in individual or collective leisure activities.

The major impediment to active and independent lives for the elderly is socially-imposed or self-imposed idleness. "Retirement," as A. M. Guillemard put it, "is the real cause of aging."

Policies and programs today

To assist the autonomous and dependent elderly, home helps are provided, but not in sufficient quantity and quality. Plans exist for coordinated health and social services within 900 catchment areas.

Priority Action Plan-15, devised by the national government, encourages localities to develop particular services, such as home helps, home meals, and laundry. These plans and programs need strong implementation.

By and large, programs are fragmented and often their objectives are compromised. For example, there is no rational policy covering employment of the elderly. Through early retirement, employers reduce staff or make room for younger workers. In the process, contributions to social security are reduced while payments are increased. Although health services are provided, policies that encourage the elderly to remain inactive and dependent are also policies that produce illness and raise service expenditures. To encourage an active life, the elderly are offered reduced prices for travel and cinema.

The year 2000

The number of elderly persons will increase, an indication that home services and financial aid will require expansion. Among the younger elderly, the needs will be less. Assuming no organized approach to problems produced by a longer span of life, costs of supporting the well elderly with pensions and the chronically ill elderly with health and social services will rise sharply. Workers will resist taxes and other financial support for the elderly.

Recommendations

1. To reduce or prevent the problems, the elderly must be provided with paid employment and other personally and socially useful activities. This may mean a system of sharing work through flexible hours. It may require abandoning retirement until well beyond age 65 for those able and willing to work. Policies to lower the retirement age must be reversed immediately.

2. Programs are needed to prepare people for retirement, to promote participation in local and national life, to strengthen family ties, and to attract retirees into organized leisure activities.

3. Policies should be adopted to prevent disease and disability and to promote healthful practices throughout the lifespan. Since old age often brings handicaps, a spectrum of supportive services – not only development of home helps and institutional services, but also types of housing suited to the elderly and permitting gradual introduction of assistance – is essential.

INDIA

The main problems today

50% of the elderly experience difficulty in maintaining an active and independent life. This problem is less for those in agricultural areas, business, professions, and higher income brackets. Poverty, unemployment, and lack of institutions for the elderly are the main causes of dependency.

Fortunately, in India, the cultural pressures are such that families still look after their aged, despite economic or other difficulties. Urbanization works against this pattern because families split up; this increases the number of old people in need of institutionalized service.

Policies and programs today

There are no clear-cut policies at the national, state, or village level designed to assist the elderly in maintaining an active and independent life.

The year 2000

Of the elderly population, now 34 million, the vast majority live in rural areas. But the culture is fast changing from agrarian to industrialized. By the year 2000, when the elderly population will have risen to over 65 million, nearly 100 cities will have a population of more than a million, as compared to ten cities today. In these large cities, unemployment, overcrowded slums, lack of sanitation, and poor housing will produce serious health problems among the elderly.

Recommendations

1. Initiate health education programs under government and voluntary agency auspices, with an emphasis on promoting positive attitudes of the elderly toward themselves, their usefulness, and the role of work in their lives.

2. Establish refresher courses in geriatrics for general practitioners.

3. Develop a cadre of health professional and paraprofessional workers who are committed to work with the elderly, and who live and work in rural areas.

4. Establish a national institute of gerontology, responsible for research and training and for managing a program of regional centers to provide job counseling, craft training, vocational guidance, and other kinds of personal assistance.

5. Revise medical education to incorporate gerontology and geriatrics in the undergraduate and postgraduate curricula.

ISRAEL

The main problems today

Only 4% of today's elderly were born in Israel. The majority immigrated in their later years and, besides problems of language and acclimatization, did not work for enough years to acquire adequate pensions. Many came from countries with lower educational and health standards, and immigrated without family.

Government and private programs designed to help the elderly function within their environment are insufficient. The income-maintenance policy is inadequate. Resources are invested disproportionately in institutional care rather than in services for the elderly living at home. Programs for health promotion and health education are minimal, and those that exist are not geared to the specific needs of the elderly. Home-care and home-help services are not fully recognized as a "right" and are not always included in the budget. Generally, the paucity of legislation defining needs, entitlements, and mandated services reflects a lack of commitment in dealing with the problems of the elderly.

No centralized machinery exists for planning and coordinating the various services for the elderly. Programs are scattered and not accessible to many of them.

Policies and programs today

The ministry of housing has ignored the specific requirements of the elderly in planning housing projects; however, a movement has started for the construction of congregate housing.

The National Insurance Law provides all elderly with a minimum income while voluntary pension systems cover a part of the elderly population.

The ministry of health actively promotes home-health care, and provides financial assistance to the major sick fund (Kupat Holim) to develop home health-care programs. Other sick funds have begun to provide limited home health-care.

Health-promotion and health-education programs are implemented by the ministry of health through neighborhood family health centers. Recognition of the need for health-education programs is growing, but the system is not yet widespread.

The year 2000

The elderly of 20 years hence will have a higher standard of living and health. They will be better educated, will have raised families in Israel, and will be better integrated into society.

However, while the total elderly population is expected to increase by about 40%, the population aged 75 and over will increase by about 60%. Because the frequency of chronic disorders and institutionalization increases substantially after the age of 75, this large increase will magnify the need for an expanded network of institutional and community-based services. If current predictions are correct, community geriatric services will not expand quickly enough to meet needs. Independent life will be more problematic for a greater percentage of the elderly.

Recommendations

1. Establish a centralized mechanism for planning and coordinating the various services for the aged.

2. Pass legislation to guarantee the elderly the right to services.

3. Develop health-education and health-promotion programs.

4. Increase the availability and variety of home-help care.

5. Emphasize preventive health services integrated into the community health and social services.

6. Encourage and coordinate mutual help groups, so that the elderly can rely to some extent on their own resources.

7. Institutionalize measures to assist local authorities, national voluntary organizations, and facilities for the elderly to expand needed services.

8. Develop programs and policies to provide secure and suitable housing.

ITALY

The main problems today

The finances of elderly people are precarious. The most acute problem for old people, housing, is in short supply and beyond their means. Many are admitted to hospital because they are homeless, or because conditions where they live are intolerable.

There are fewer, if any, children and grandchildren to help the aged. Outsiders willing to help are hard to find, even if offered payment.

Serious mental health problems among the elderly reflect lack of preparation for old age, resulting, for example, in the loss of social role.

Cultural traditions disadvantage elderly women. They tend to live longer, are unable to be financially independent, and have no interests of their own. However, this situation is bound to improve.

Policies and programs today

The Italian Constitution calls for equality among citizens, health care, and assistance to the disabled. A national health service is established by law. Regional laws exist on assistance to the aged. However, there do not seem to be any well-defined policies or programs to implement these objectives.

The National Health Plan provides for special attention to the elderly, but this has not been translated into a specified goal or strategy. The government's ability to carry out well-designed programs is doubted. More likely to be effective are efforts to inform the public of the problems of the elderly through the mass media; to encourage the elderly to take up an activity, be it no more than a hobby; and to alter the role of elderly women in the family, as regards housekeeping and child-minding.

The year 2000

Problems of social welfare will be even more acute, particularly in large cities. There will be enormous problems in providing assistance to the disabled and to people unable to support themselves. Fewer people of working age will be available to support elders, who will comprise over 22% of the total population. However, the higher educational levels of the self-supporting (particularly women) are expected to improve this picture to some extent.

Recommendations

1. Encourage and help people to stay in good physical and mental health for as long as possible.

2. Delay the transition from an active to an inactive life for as long as possible.

3. Integrate retirees into productive activities through training programs.

JAPAN

The main problems today

Because of age discrimination in employment, older workers (including those who "retire" at age 55) lose social position, self-confidence, and willingness to keep their skills and knowledge up to date. Among other problems are: increased medical care expenses for the elderly, increased number of bedridden elderly (about 400,000 in 1979), high rate of suicide among the elderly, and an increase in the number of elderly individuals and couples living alone.

The elderly population in Japan, and the proportion of elderly in the population, are increasing rapidly.

Policies and programs today

Programs exist for free health education for the elderly, free medical examination, free medical care for those aged 70 and over, and free rehabilitation. Participation in these programs is highly encouraged. A variety of facilities for the elderly exist, including public nursing homes for the needy (70,000 beds in 903 establishments in 1979), public and private homes and low-cost housing (11,000 capacity in 1979), welfare centers (853 in 1978), and club houses (2,346 in 1978). Residents in public homes for the elderly pay according to family ability. The public facilities are supervised by local government, under central government plans.

The year 2000

Providing for the growing population aged 75 and over will be difficult. Medical care expenses will increase greatly as those aged 60 and over grow to over 20% of the total population. The number of elderly who are bedridden and afflicted with senile dementia may increase sharply. However, circulatory and rheumatic disorders surely will decrease as a result of improvements in therapy and lifestyle, particularly exercise and nutritional habits. Some types of cancer may become preventable.

Recommendations

1. To help counteract misconceptions about the elderly, conduct scientific studies of ability to work at different stages of adult life. Conduct studies on methods of rehabilitating people for work.

2. Reform and make comprehensive the health-care and health-insurance systems (public and private) so that:

- Comprehensive health services are offered, including health education, health promotion (such as physical fitness), rehabilitation, and disease prevention (especially hypertension control).
- Public and private insurance are coordinated or unified, so that benefit packages and reimbursement approaches are comprehensive and standardized.

39

- More geriatrically-oriented personnel are trained, such as home helps, public health nurses, social workers, paramedical aides, and physicians.

- Day-care, short-stay hospital, and primary-care medical services tailored to the elderly are developed and more nursing homes are established.

3. Increase spending on geriatric research.

4. Incorporate volunteer activities as part of schooling and adult life, beginning in schools and continuing into old age.

KENYA

The main problems today

The basic problem is lack of community awareness of the needs of the elderly. Facilities that could be provided for them are lacking, such as old people's homes and other housing. No organization trained in services for older people exists. The elderly tend to be isolated, poorly fed, and dependent on the extended family.

Policies and programs today

The country lacks general policies for the elderly. They have to depend somewhat on traditional ties, whose continuity is questionable.

The year 2000

Problems will get worse owing to breakdown of the extended family. As the number of elderly grows, increases are expected in fractures and other disorders of locomotion, and in mental illness.

Recommendations

1. Create community services.

2. Re-evaluate and reform health-care policies to meet changes expected by 2000, including more geriatric facilities and personnel to deal with the elderly population.

3. Provide facilities for retirement.

NIGERIA

The main problems today

There is a lack of adequate and accessible health care, housing, transport, adult and vocational education, recreation clubs, and other social facilities.

Policies and programs today

According to the Constitution, "the State shall direct its policy toward ensuring ... that suitable ... old-age care and pensions ... are provided for all citizens." The fourth National Development Plan (1981–85) states the intention of providing for the care of the elderly, including the creation of old-age homes. The extent to which this will be carried out remains to be seen.

Policies and programs for social and community development will benefit the elderly in due course. Among these are the basic health services scheme, government housing schemes, and nutrition, adult literacy, water supply, and sanitation programs. These will raise the standard of living and health of the community, equipping people to cope better with life when they become elderly.

The year 2000

Today's problems will worsen, in view of the expected 95% rise in total population, 106% rise in population aged 60 and over, and larger migration to the cities. Lack of family planning will impede development of healthier, better educated, and more socially responsible families, which would be more likely to take care of the elderly.

Recommendations

1. Maintain and extend the custom by which elders retain some of their traditional role in society, even after retirement.

2. Incorporate elements about aging in mass literacy campaigns and at all levels of the educational system.

3. Ensure balanced and decentralized rural development to strengthen rural society, including elderly members.

4. Establish more realistic planning and organization of health and social service programs, with a role for public participation.

PHILIPPINES

The main problems today

Because of unemployment and other reasons for insufficient income, a reasonable living standard, including decent housing, cannot be maintained.

Health-care facilities, for example geriatric clinics, are scarce, particularly in rural areas.

Feelings of loneliness and isolation due to increasing physical weakness are common. Social values and attitudes towards the elderly are changing for the worse as a result of urbanization and modernization.

Policies and programs today

Government employees get retirement pensions after the compulsory retirement age of 65, or at age 60 after at least 15 years of service. Upon retirement, a lump sum equivalent to five years' salary is given. After five years, the retiree gets a pension for life. Private employees have social security retirement benefits similar to those of government employees.

Medicare (government health insurance) benefits are extended to both government and private employees.

None of the above programs apply to the unemployed or self-employed.

Programs and services, available to a small fraction of the elderly, include:

– A nutrition program under the ministry of health, emphasizing proper nutritional needs.

– Adult education programs, in day centers for the elderly and residential facilities, run by the ministry of social services and development and voluntary organizations.

– City and town health centers, for the medical needs of the elderly in urban and rural areas.

– Symposia and seminars through organized senior citizens' clubs and organizations, as well as discussions by the elderly on common issues, problems, and concerns.

– Employment opportunities, including sheltered placements, and help in starting small businesses (a self-employment assistance program, providing interest-free loans, run by the ministry of social services and development).

The year 2000

Rural areas will have a higher proportion of elderly due to migration of young workers to urban areas. Housing problems will worsen.

Recommendations

1. Accelerate rural development programs (including electrification and road construction) to produce more jobs and industries, in the hope of deterring the younger population from migrating to urban areas.

2. Establish rooming units for the elderly, to enable them to stay close to their families.

3 Offer pre-retirement planning and counseling (including investment counseling as retirement benefits improve) to government and private employees.

4. Provide jobs for the skilled elderly who are still able to work.

POLAND

The main problems today

The maintenance of a normal life depends on physical, material, and social independence. For most retired Poles, the main problem is inadequate income.

Among people over 60 years of age, about 30% are healthy and require no special help, whereas among those aged 75 years or more only about 15% are independent and require no special care. However, health services and social services do not always reach out to old people. Nor are they coordinated effectively.

There are no health maintenance or preventive geriatric services for those who are well. Care of persons with chronic disease is unsatisfactory because beds, nurses, and transport facilities are inadequate. This leads to over-dependence of the sick elderly on their younger household members and neighbors.

Policies and programs today

For those lacking a regular, adequate income or money to weather a crisis, arrangements for financial help may be initiated by medical workers.

Limits on work by retired persons are being decreased.

A system of free medical care covers all persons over retirement age (generally 60 years for women and 65 for men), including free medicines, hospitalization, and sanitaria. Home care of people with chronic diseases is performed by visiting nurses, including Polish Red Cross nurses. There is a training program in geriatrics for nurses and social workers, but not for medical students generally.

Social policy emphasizes aid to families and to old people within families. To support this orientation in policy, the Council for Family Affairs, an official advisory body, came into being in 1979.

The year 2000

The number of bedridden elderly people with chronic diseases, requiring constant and well-organized medical and social care, will increase. The number of old people living in isolation from younger members of the family will also increase, but standards of independent living will be higher because of higher aspirations.

Ensuring independence, and providing facilities for old people so that they can remain in their habitual environment, will depend on the situation of an old person in his or her family and on the benefits, especially services, which can be provided by society. Old people will be able to select a place of residence close to their children, either with a family, in homes for retired persons, or in homes of social help. There will be universal access to geriatric rehabilitation wards, health centers, and health resorts, enabling revitalization of elderly people.

In certain occupations, such as those in health and social services for the elderly, there will be opportunities for paid employment for the elderly.

Recommendations

1. By removing financial, organizational, and attitudinal barriers:

− Create a system of integrated medical and social care.

− Extend care of a sick and physically infirm person to his or her own home.

− Prepare systematically for old age, from a medical and psychological point of view.

2. Introduce active medical care, including periodic check-ups with treatment if necessary, for people over 70 or 75.

3. Through research, well-aged clinics, and rehabilitation services, develop and apply preventive geriatrics and rehabilitation.

SWEDEN

The main problems today

Swedes believe, erroneously, that the elderly tend naturally to be inactive and should live a passive life. Aging is often considered equivalent to illness. But many old people actually desire and need physical, intellectual, and emotional activity. The elderly have capacities to contribute constructively to society, but they remain idle.

Swedish society produces isolation for many of the elderly. They live alone in their homes or apartments. This isolation impedes participation in meaningful activities, which are important factors in physical and mental well-being. Those aged 80 years and older are particularly isolated and at risk of being unable to meet their physical and mental needs, and thus of becoming ill and requiring care.

Many elderly do not seek medical advice for curable diseases. Doctors and patients may confuse manifestations of aging with disease, resulting either in unnecessary treatment or in delay of necessary treatment.

Policies and programs today

Sweden has well-developed systems of income maintenance and social services.

Scientific knowledge of the elderly is being accumulated. Eventually, this will produce better knowledge of the elderly as a resource, their real medical and social needs for assistance, and means of preventing or postponing the consequences of aging and illness.

University-level training in gerontology makes possible improved research and service.

The year 2000

The elderly will comprise about 22% of the entire population. Because the increase will be greatest for the group above 80 years, demand for social care and health care will grow substantially. In a stagnating economy, the allocation of further resources to meet such demand may not be possible.

A tendency towards over-diagnosis and unnecessary therapy, due to difficulties in differentiating between aging and disease, will persist.

Trends in lifestyle and socio-environmental factors (such as inactivity, malnutrition, and social isolation) may raise morbidity rates within older age groups. This is especially true for women, whose tobacco and alcohol habits will come to resemble those of men.

Recommendations

1. Expand efforts to increase knowledge of differences between disease and normal aging and its consequences.

2. Promote scientific studies to lay the basis for intervention, to enhance quality of life among the elderly, and to reduce negative consequences of aging.

3. Establish information and education programs to combat prejudices against aging.

4. Re-structure geriatric care, to achieve a system which is able to draw on a spectrum of services to meet individual needs.

UNITED KINGDOM

The main problems today

1. Attitudinal: persuading people that long life is the norm, and that retirement is not a lucky bonus for a few but the prerogative of many. Lack of esteem and self-worth. Lack of incentives among the socially disadvantaged to maintain activity and independence.

2. Health: personal behavior that damages health (such as smoking, alcohol, lack of exercise, and poor nutrition). Primary-care teams are inappropriately trained and oriented.

3. Social and economic: income deficiencies. Inadequate housing and transport. Less-than-optimal deployment of social resources. Too few domiciliary services.

Policies and programs today

The National Health Service (NHS) provides free medical care. Specialist medical services for the elderly have become an accepted part of the NHS hospital services in the past 20 years. Domiciliary care is provided partly by NHS general practitioners, partly by voluntary services (such as "meals on wheels"), and partly by local authority financed health visitors and social workers. The NHS also provides specific services such as chiropody.

The government financed Health Education Council concentrates mainly on propaganda against smoking and alcohol. The department of health has a research program on the health problems of the elderly.

The government provides a state pension and other means-tested benefits, including help with rent, rates, and fuel costs. Local authorities provide sheltered housing and grants for home improvements. Housing associations help promote home ownership among the poorer sections of society. Local government may also provide free (or cheap) transport for the elderly.

The year 2000

Present problems will continue. Demographic changes could mean that 20% of citizens – those in retirement – have a negative view of their potential, with resultant stresses on the rest of the population.

On the other hand, there should be more surviving couples as compared to bereaved and childless individuals, so reducing the problems of loneliness and isolation.

Recommendations

1. Attitudinal:

- Conduct a massive public relations campaign aimed at reversing stereotypes of aging.
- Emphasize correct perspectives through health-education and adult-education agencies, and in pre-retirement courses.

2. Health:

- Initiate a government-sponsored program for education on healthy behavior.
- Re-orient the primary-care system toward unified social and health care and toward prevention, with abolition of fee-for-service payment of general practitioners.
- Improve support of research.

3. Social and economic:

- Index all pensions, state and occupational, to maintain purchasing power in the face of inflation.
- Produce more adapted or purpose-built housing, to cope with changing needs of the elderly person.
- Improve the flexibility and accessibility of surface transport and improve pedestrian facilities.

- Shift resources from institutions to ambulatory and domiciliary services, *not* from the public sector of the economy to the private sector.

- Broaden the role of the trade unions in seeking pensions, retirement education, job-sharing, and sabbatical approaches to the work load.

- Encourage phased retirement.

UNITED STATES OF AMERICA

The main problems today

A sizeable proportion of elderly Americans – especially in later old age – suffer from multiple economic, socio-environmental, and health deficits. They may lack primary health care and a socially-supportive environment of family, informal helpers, and formal social services. Many experience environmental isolation. They may lack access to adequate, affordable transportation. They may live in surroundings filled with architectural barriers and bristling with physical threats. Given the increasing prevalence with age of chronic physical and mental disabilities – not only heart, rheumatic, vision, and hearing disorders but also depression and senile dementia – life in the circumstances described above is all too often bleak and unfulfilling.

For the well elderly who wish to work or otherwise play roles as active producers and contributors to society, opportunities may be severely limited. It may be easier to accept a role as a passive receiver and consumer.

Policies and programs today

The preamble to the federal Older Americans Act specifies independence in later life as a national goal. Under this act, Administration on Aging programs ostensibly are directed to encouraging activity and independence, through such means as senior centers, meals-on-wheels, and congregate dining and transport services. There are federal programs to encourage voluntarism among older persons. Voluntary agencies offer services to, and occupations for, the elderly.

There are public and private pension programs and government regulation of pensions. Income is provided on the basis of age or poverty status through public welfare programs, such as Supplemental Security Income, food stamps, and housing subsidies.

Public programs that pay for medical and hospital care exist as a part of social insurance (Medicare), social welfare for the poor (Medicaid), and veterans benefits. Federal health efforts include special disease-control programs. Programs designed to move geriatrics from a custodial mode to a preventive, maintenance, or rehabilitation mode are scarce. Disability benefits are available through public and private organizations.

Federal support has been directed toward research on the causes and treatment of senile dementia.

The year 2000

Many elderly people will be dependent and will lack an adequate income. There will be growing resentment of the elderly by the younger population and a steady erosion of family support. However, health maintenance and rehabilitation probably will improve.

Recommendations

1. Re-structure income maintenance policies to ensure adequate retirement income.

2. Provide financial incentives for family care of older persons.

3. Improve the organization of volunteer services, including many more elderly volunteers, and their integration with smaller numbers of paid personnel, who would include retirees. Use the elderly to greater advantage in caring for the elderly.

4. Establish delayed, flexible, and phased retirement.

5. Provide greater training and job opportunities for older workers.

6. Develop a private market for supportive services.

7. Develop better living environments for older people.

8. Organize a major expansion of self-help programs.

9. Provide for greater local control of programs.

10. Foster the adoption of improved lifestyles (diet, smoking, use of alcohol, etc.) by adults including those, now middle-aged, who will be elderly by the year 2000.

ROUND ONE

(replies by topic)

Chapter 1

COPING WITH CHRONIC PHYSICAL AND MENTAL PROBLEMS

Order of priority given to "Health":

1	AUSTRALIA	BRAZIL	JAPAN	PHILIPPINES	POLAND	SWEDEN
2	W GERMANY	USA				
3	EGYPT	INDIA	UK			
4	ISRAEL	ITALY	KENYA			
5	NIGERIA					
6						
7	FRANCE					
8						
9						

The main problems today

Most older people develop some degree of chronic physical, emotional, or mental illness. Yet a major worldwide shortage exists of trained health professionals and facilities for the treatment and care of chronically ill individuals, according to the experts contacted in the Sandoz Institute study.

The experts listed the following as major health problems of the elderly:

Heart diseases
Cerebrovascular diseases
Cancer
Depression and senile dementia
Arthritis
Orthopedic problems (including osteoporosis and hip fractures)
Diminished or lost hearing and/or vision
Dental problems.

A representative national pattern of age-related disease is seen in that offered by Australian experts. Studies showed that a third of older Australians die of heart disease, about 20% of cancer, and about 13% of cerebrovascular diseases. The proportion of persons suffering from at least one chronic condition rises steadily with age. About 50% of those aged 25 to 44 have a chronic condition, while over 80% of those 75 years of age and older have at least one.

Respondents in the study cite lifelong poor housing, poor nutrition, inadequate health care, lack of emergency medicine, and environmental toxins as contributing factors to such chronic health problems. Swedish experts emphasize widowhood as a risk factor. The Italians add "marginalization", loss of social role, lack of interests, and inactivity. A fatalistic attitude toward chronic disease is considered a risk factor by various experts.

In Brazil, the experts report, many older people are living in conditions "inconsistent with dignity". Experts from Kenya report malnutrition among their elderly. Many countries report undernutrition.

In affluent countries, many factors combine to make it difficult for the elderly to be well nourished: dental problems, isolation, lack of pleasure in eating, poverty, and other barriers to obtaining food. All of these factors contribute to what is known in the United States as the "tea and toast" syndrome.

Almost global difficulty exists in meeting the health needs of the elderly. Experts listed such obstacles as a general ignorance about treating and preventing diseases frequent in old age, and a dearth of trained care-givers, especially geriatric personnel. Some countries, such as Nigeria, face special problems of integrating "traditional healers" into their long-term care system. Most countries would like to encourage private citizens and volunteers to become involved in helping the elderly obtain medical care. Polish experts report an intensive effort to train visiting nurses and social workers to help meet this growing need.

Geriatric medicine appears to be universally underdeveloped. West German experts report that many doctors lack knowledge of the diseases common in old age. Superficial examinations lead to erroneous or partial diagnoses; for example, "senile dementia" is given as a diagnosis without any effort to rule out infection, drug reaction, or other acute and reversible illness. This is a complaint voiced by experts in the US and other countries. Japanese experts report a shortage of trained personnel and an over-emphasis on acute care to the neglect of chronic care.

"Enormous price tags have been placed on medical care," according to US experts. Yet, insurance coverage is maldesigned for the elderly – not covering preventive or chronic care at times, and often not paying for needed items such as dentures. Iatrogenic or practitioner-caused illness is considered by the experts to be far too common in the US, and drugs in general are not well managed. The typical elderly American is on multiple medications – up to about 13 at any one time.

Other problems:

– In France only school-age children are screened for illness, not the highly vulnerable elderly.

– In Japan, experts would like to see a better linkage of medical care with social welfare and educational programs.

– Kenya has only 2,000 beds for the chronically ill of all ages.

– In Poland, more beds are needed for the chronically ill.

– Nigeria reports inadequate health-care services of all sorts.

– In Egypt, experts report a lack of mental health services despite the fact that chronic depression is a major health problem among the elderly.

Policies and programs today

Cultural values, as well as financial resources, shape the provision of care for the chronically ill elderly. In the developing countries, necessity and tradition have largely left such care to families; in the developed countries, there are more, but seldom enough, trained professionals and facilities.

Screening for disease, or conditions likely to produce or aggravate disease, is widely considered to be important in preventing illness. Experts from France report a few successful centers of disease prevention for the elderly. In Poland, all medical services for the elderly are free and various appliances, such as dentures, hearing aids, and glasses, are provided.

In Japan, older people are entitled to a free annual check-up. While acknowledging that senile dementia is a major problem there, and one that has been largely neglected, Japanese experts voiced the opinion that the elderly sometimes exhibit authoritarian or rigid behavior patterns, a tendency that complicates care for their mental disorders. Hip fractures, largely due to osteoporosis, are a serious problem, causing a third of all surgical operations in older Japanese.

Education about health hazards is valued as the key to limiting some chronic disorders, such as lung cancer. Sweden has an active program to educate the public about the harmful effects of tobacco and alcohol. Australia, too, has such a campaign and adds to it information about poor diets, stress, and lack of exercise. Japan is trying to teach its citizens about diet, emphasizing the health risks – particularly hypertension – associated with a salty diet.

An intensive effort to diagnose, and if possible prevent, disease throughout life is seen in West Germany. The view that the health of the baby to an extent determines health in later life is a foundation of the West German program. It embraces a broad array of preventive and screening measures, including: tests for tuberculosis and cancer, prenatal care, infant and baby clinics, monitoring of work-places and restaurants for sanitation and safety, vaccination programs, and genetic counseling.

Israel provides general health services for ambulatory patients, paid for by a variety of private and government programs. Most dental services are private, but a few subsidized clinics for the elderly exist. The government is developing a policy of early detection, but admits that specialized geriatric services are underdeveloped.

The geriatric center at Alexandria University, Egypt, offers training to a limited number of nurses. The elderly can receive eyeglasses, hearing aids, etc. under the medical insurance program, but to date few elderly are covered.

In Nigeria, federal government programs give special attention to orthopedic and neuropsychiatric programs. WHO collaborating centers are being set up in Lagos and Aro.

In France, day-care centers were opened and then scrapped before conclusions could be drawn about their effectiveness and drawbacks. Home-care services are promoted, but the way in which the patient's financial contribution is fixed, the pressure groups formed by independent nurses, and arbitrary decisions taken by regional health insurance funds are said to impede their development.

The year 2000

The "old" old – aged 80 and over – will be a much larger group in the year 2000. Many more people will suffer chronic diseases, including senile dementia, arthritis, cancer, and cerebrovascular disorders. On the other hand, by virtue of numbers there will be more healthy older people, and by and large the older generation will be a better educated and healthier one.

Responses to the study range from very pessimistic to quite positive. On the one hand, experts from Italy expect to see more "alienation" and hence more alcohol and drug abuse. On the other hand, experts in Australia expect improved diagnostic and treatment methods and more advanced organ replacements yielding a healthier group.

Experts in most countries expect a severe taxing of already over-stretched social and medical facilities. Kenyan experts foresee mental deterioration from lack of adequate shelter, food, clothing, and security.

In Israel, India, and the UK, even if the health of the elderly population improves, economic capacities may not stretch sufficiently to cover those needing services.

Italian experts fear that environmental toxins will generate rising rates of cancer, and that urbanization will bring more disintegration of the family, loneliness, and alienation, factors that promote institutionalization.

Optimistic notes are sounded by Australian and French experts. They anticipate that progress in medical research and improved personal habits will yield a healthier aged population. People will stop smoking, eat more appropriately, continue to exercise, and learn better ways to handle emotional stress.

There is almost complete discouragement on the subject of senile dementia. None of the experts believe that researchers are anywhere near to understanding the causes. They are therefore gloomy about the possibilities of preventives or cures. They expect today's prevalence rates to continue, a prospect that would mean – in the context of less morbidity and mortality from other diseases – a rising population of demented individuals for whom care will be needed.

Swedish experts point out that unless the life expectancy of men improves soon, the year 2000 could bring an increasing number of widows – lonely, depressed, and in need of institutional services. Sweden expects a 37% increase in the number of people aged 80 and older by the year 2000.

Israeli experts believe the social support system in the community will be inadequate to meet the needs. The demand for institutional services will increase for this reason, as well as because of an absolute increase of individuals past age 80.

Recommendations

More research on geriatric diseases is recommended by an overwhelming majority of the international experts. They reiterate that research is necessary to establish effective programs of prevention and treatment of chronic diseases. US experts insist that the highest research priorities should go to senile dementia. Less effort should go to prolongation of life. Rather, they say, efforts should be directed to "squaring the disability curve", that is, shortening the period of illness and disability at the end of life.

Programs of health maintenance through self-help, and organized programs of prevention, are highly recommended. Public education via the mass media and schools is emphasized. UK experts argue for strong programs against smoking cigarettes and drinking alcoholic beverages. Their objectives include attacks on the industries that profit from these commodities.

Many experts say the elderly must participate in maintaining their own health. Learning about the long-range value of personal hygiene, proper diet, and exercise is essential to maximizing the opportunity for good health in old age. The elderly must be taught to seek medical help in a timely fashion. The West Germans would include education about being an active and constructive partner in one's own medical care. From India comes the suggestion that health-education programs in high schools teach elementary nursing, first aid, and nutrition.

Self-help, reliance on the family and community, and assistance in a medical crisis to enable an older person to stay at home are all viewed as desirable. Nigeria, Kenya, and India – where institutional services for the elderly are lacking – all stress that the individual, the family, and the community must work together to care for older persons with chronic diseases.

Nurses and doctors trained in geriatrics are needed, according to all the experts. Nigerian, Kenyan, Israeli, and US experts urge that paraprofessionals be trained to work with the geriatric population.

All sorts of facilities for the elderly are needed throughout the world. Kenya needs community institutions. Japan would like a range of facilities, including geriatric hospitals and a network of nursing homes with 20–50 beds. These nursing homes would be annexed to general hospitals.

To make the best use of facilities, Australian experts suggest that "priority review" committees be established; they would decide which patients are entitled to which services, and whether services are used wisely. Experts from India advise a national program to help the elderly.

By nation, here are capsule recommendations on various topics:

From Italy:

Establish more sensitive regulation of the environment, so the elderly can get about safely and easily to participate in social activities, leisure and recreational pursuits, and family or social exchanges. Promote a cleaner environment, more natural foodstuffs, and places for relaxation. Ban smoking in all public places. Reduce the competitiveness of society to alleviate stress and attendant disorders. Intensify research into mental aging. Provide preventive medicine for the middle-aged.

From Egypt:

Promote visits to the partially or seriously disabled elderly by nurses, social workers, and volunteers so as to lessen isolation and furnish assistance in independent living.

From Sweden:

Design and adjust housing and traffic patterns to accommodate the functional capacities of the elderly, thus promoting their mobility, comfort, and participation in community activities. Organize support for the bereaved person. Simply as a matter of maintaining physical and mental health, accord the vigorous elderly opportunities to continue in their occupations.

From Israel:

Educate physicians to take an active, rather than fatalistic, approach to care of the aging. Develop programs of disease prevention and health promotion directed at improving lifelong habits of nutrition, exercise, and avoidance of toxic materials.

From France:

Protect workers against occupational hazards. Guard the environment against water and air pollution. Train all professional caregivers in geriatrics, especially the inter-relationships of somatic, psychological, social, and economic conditions and philosophical outlooks. Encourage physical activity and yearly check-ups, with follow-up of risk factors, especially hypertension.

From Poland:

Raise living standards. Emphasize preventive geriatrics.

From West Germany:

Make health promotion campaigns more effective by improving doctor-patient rapport, especially through more time for discussion during office visits. Because periodic check-ups by a physician are not cost-effective, emphasize screening and other disease-prevention measures. Disseminate information on drugs in language patients can understand.

From the US:

Alter medical education to emphasize functional assessment of the patient and treatment based on it. Change reimbursement incentives to favor time spent with patients and good treatment results, as opposed to paying for procedures. Encourage and teach self-help and peer support.

From the UK:

Establish a national institute of gerontology to study chronic disabling conditions of the elderly. Undertake aggressive state action against tobacco use. Shape the environment and improve transport to permit access to shops and sites for leisure activities.

From India:

Promote undergraduate, postgraduate, and continuing education of doctors in geriatrics. Through the mass media and public meetings, educate people about healthy lifelong habits.

From Japan:

Prepare and disseminate to the public information on handling personal issues of aging, such as development of leisure-time activities. Inform the public of concepts and models of successful aging as they are identified.

From Kenya:

Provide good comprehensive and social care.

From the Philippines:

Establish a geriatric section in every hospital. Train geriatric specialists.

From Brazil:

"Look after each and every individual."

Chapter 2
ENSURING SUITABLE HOUSING

Order of priority given to "Housing":

1	ITALY			
2	UK			
3	AUSTRALIA	W. GERMANY	ISRAEL	KENYA
4	NIGERIA	USA		
5	FRANCE	PHILIPPINES	POLAND	
6	BRAZIL	INDIA	SWEDEN	
7	EGYPT	JAPAN		
8				
9				

The main problems today

Overview

Enabling the elderly to remain in their homes as long as possible appears to be an almost universal goal. However, many of the world's elders have never owned their own home and have never had a separate residence. Many live with families through most of their mature lives, as head of household and later as dependant. This is almost always the case in less developed countries, reflecting widespread housing shortages. In Brazil, Kenya, India, the Philippines, and other nations, an urgent priority is improved housing for all. In these countries, the hope is that the elderly will benefit as the general need is addressed. In the more developed countries, the problems of suitable housing for the elderly emphasize their particular characteristics and needs.

In all the surveyed countries, the elderly tend to live in poor housing. In less developed countries, they have elementary needs for a secure roof and potable water. In the more developed countries, they tend to occupy the oldest and most deteriorated houses, which may jeopardize their health and survival.

The issue of suitable housing merges with other issues which, discussed in detail in other chapters, are simply noted in passing here. Housing may be the physical embodiment of poverty, relation-ships with younger family members, and relationships with the community and society at large. A dwelling may be run-down be-cause the occupant lacks income to make repairs, or to move to housing that is more suitable to his or her stage of dependency, or because of need for proximity to services. Housing may be too small to permit a family headed by a younger adult to incorporate aged parents or relatives. This in itself may disrupt — in the context of population shifts due to urbanization and industrialization — tradi-tional patterns of family life. The disruption may bring emotional upset and even mental illness.

The ability of a chronically ill aged person to live independently may be restricted by lack of local supportive services, especially home-delivered health, social, and chore services. This absence may, eventually and prematurely, force re-location to a hospital, nursing home, hostel, or congregate-living facility, if any are available. The search for inexpensive quarters may concentrate the poor elderly into slums, expose them to disease and crime, and isolate or segre-gate them from society at large. The wealthy elderly may choose privately developed communities, but these individuals may not escape difficulties attached to the aging population around them and the needs and costs of community services. Whether rich or poor, elderly persons face the probability that, over time, suitable housing will become unsuitable because mobility and other abilities for self-care may change. Only recently has thought been given to housing design that is adaptable to changing circumstances, so that the aged individual need not change residence.

The experts responding to the Sandoz Institute survey point out that costs of maintaining a dwelling often become prohibitive on a declining old-age income. Older people may be permanently dis-placed because there are no services available to tide them over an emergency, or temporary incapacity, in their own homes. At times, older people who would benefit from living in a smaller dwelling, or one without barriers to getting around, or that is less conducive to falls and other accidents, cannot move because of the expense of doing so or the price of other, especially newer, housing. Indeed, they may become prisoners of inflation, urbanization, construction costs, and other factors that push up the price of suitable housing.

Housing problems of the elderly overlap housing problems of their adult children. The very increases in costs of living that prompt conjoint living may intensify inter-family tensions. If an aged and sick parent is accommodated, the parent's care and supervision may add to stresses on younger women in the family who, while retaining home-maker responsibility, have to find paid work. The double burden adds to conflicts over authority between young and old. In Egypt, for example, the elderly living with adult children often criticize the younger women for having abandoned traditional roles to go to work. However, it is also true that an aged parent may contribute money and labor to the running of a household.

Urban change

When younger persons re-locate to find work or higher wages, not only are older people left behind but the young are deprived of the assistance the elderly could give. Sometimes, the elders are left behind in deteriorating cities, the Italian experts report. In Egypt, Poland, and Nigeria, young people emigrate to cities and the elderly remain in isolated rural areas. In Sweden, the elderly are left in city neighborhoods, living in old tenements that lack elevators. In France, many elders live in condemned buildings.

Urban development may change a neighborhood's character to something less convenient and friendly than before. In France, the introduction of supermarkets has changed the traditional pattern of small neighborhood shops. In Sweden, new highways have made some neighborhoods unsafe for the elderly.

In less developed countries such as Brazil, Kenya, Nigeria, and the Philippines, the elderly often live in slums or squatter villages. In Kenya, obtaining ventilation via doors or windows is a problem; many houses are made of mud and have thatched roofs, and consequently are quick to deteriorate during the rainy season. Indian experts report that the elderly in their country often have no choice other than to live with their families, often in overcrowded conditions, until they die.

Rural areas throughout the world offer far fewer services than do urban ones. In Poland, although the urban elderly are said to live well enough, the village elderly almost always are in old wooden houses without running water or toilets. In the UK, many older people need subsidies to repair their homes. Ironically, renovations financed by subsidies to landlords tend to make housing more attractive and produce higher rents, which the elderly often cannot afford.

Policies and programs today

Throughout the world, housing policy is shaped by diverse factors – history, philosophy, tradition, and demography as well as finances and technology. It is traditional in India for the elderly to remain with their families. Supporting them is considered a bound duty of any physically fit son. Family ties are so strong that separation may cause deep emotional upset. The government, despite financial limitations, offers the elderly a subsidy which they may contribute to the family income.

In Sweden, national economic trends have led to curtailment in housing benefits for the elderly.

Housing policy in Israel recognizes that the demography of today's and tomorrow's elderly will differ. Today's population was formed largely by immigrants. Their needs and cultural diversity are reflected in housing policy. At the same time, policy-makers must consider a marked trend away from life in extended family units and the fact that many older Israelis inhabit deteriorated buildings, hastily put up at the time the country was formed. To serve the elderly without uprooting them, the government plans to renovate this housing.

The UK exemplifies a country with a variety of housing options. Communities traditionally have offered sheltered housing under supervision of a warden. In a contemporary adaptation, a mobile warden offers assistance to older people in their own homes. The government funds older home-owners so they can make repairs. As in other countries, volunteer groups may offer repair service. Some communities offer home helps, individuals who perform domestic services for the elderly with disabilities. Communities also provide home-delivered meals and sponsor community lunch groups as well as telephones, crutches, and other supports to the elderly living in their own homes.

Australia has innovated the "granny flat". This small, mobile unit, installed inexpensively at the back of a home property, houses one or two people. They live independently while having family contact. This concept is being applied in the US and the UK.

Hostels – facilities with bed-sitting rooms and communal dining facilities – are popular in Australia, often run by religious organizations. Generally, taking up residence in a hostel demands a lump-sum payment upon admission and weekly payments to cover the ongoing expenses. Australia also has a program to assist families who care for relatives who would otherwise be institutionalized. (A benefit payment of about $3 a day was current in September 1980.)

Experts from West Germany report a multiplicity of services and types of housing available to the elderly. Among services are meals on wheels, home help, personal assistance (bathing, etc.), shopping, counseling, visiting, escort and wheelchair provision, home cleaning, excursions, mobile libraries, senior centers, rehabilitation and occupational therapy, sports and recreational programs, and provision of work saving appliances and clothing.

Americans have a variety of types of housing, ranging from publicly-subsidized housing to privately-financed retirement communities. The distribution of options across the country is highly uneven. No unified national policy on housing for the aged exists. Some US communities offer many supportive services. Some offer little. Rural communities tend to be the most deprived.

The French have developed a variety of options. One concept, *foyer soleil*, involves a complex of apartment buildings with restaurants, shops, and other facilities nearby. The hostel concept described by the Australians is also popular in France. Experts in France report a concern for avoiding age-segregation. Where the French elderly have stable support from families, neighbors, and social services, they are more likely to avoid institutionalization. Telephones are considered important to maintaining independence and should be installed as needed.

For the Polish elderly, special houses are available in some cities for temporary visits, and there are homes for the bedridden or retired elderly. A few supportive services such as domestic help are available.

Financial incentives

Tax relief for elderly home-owners or for those who care for them are common. The elderly in the US and India, for instance, receive tax concessions. The Japanese contemplate special tax exemptions and inheritance tax advantages for adults who care for elderly parents. Australia has programs to help the elderly find and keep housing. Cash assistance is given to some older renters, and tax reductions to older home-owners.

Nigeria provides some federal and state mortgage assistance. Israel offers government financial loans to overcrowded families, sponsors a neighborhood renewal program which both constructs new houses and converts buildings to residences, and offers a means-tested program to provide supplemental income and rent assistance.

Sometimes it is neither the state nor the family, but the employers, who step in to ensure suitable housing. In Nigeria, a country with a severe housing shortage, some companies and banks have built housing for their employees. A small proportion of well-to-do employees have access to company-subsidized housing and may retain the homes after retirement. However government employees, provided with homes as perquisites of their positions, lose the homes at retirement. In India, a few industrial organizations have helped employees build cooperative housing, in which older people may live as dependents.

Supplementary services

In West Germany, India, Australia, Israel, the UK, Sweden, France, Italy, Israel, and the US, the elderly are encouraged to volunteer to help other older persons in ways that support independent living. Japan, which has no tradition of volunteer services, is attempting to build one. The Philippines are without volunteers. The Egyptian government is allocating free or low-price housing to voluntary organizations working with the elderly.

Poland is trying to develop a cadre of trained social workers to travel and coordinate services for the elderly throughout the country. Visiting nurses are being trained to care for mentally and physically disabled persons who are home-bound.

The year 2000

Housing prospects for the elderly in the year 2000 look bleak. Experts predict a worsening of today's problems. Despite an 18-year lead time and despite widespread awareness of problems and needs, all predictions are dire.

In Italy, the expected rise in the elderly population probably will make it harder to serve them. Inflation, particularly in fuel costs, may preclude provision of better housing. Indian experts expect that the growing numbers of the elderly will intensify the inter-generational struggle for goods and services. Urban slums may spread in India and the Philippines; many older people will be living as squatters.

West German experts expect more difficulty in financing home-delivered services. They foresee two generations in retirement by the year 2000.

The US experts fear that increased costs of building homes, transportation, goods, and services may isolate the elderly. Because young people will migrate to the "Sunbelt" states of the south and south-west to find jobs, older relatives will be left behind in northern cities. This could magnify institutionalization of the elderly – the most expensive housing solution. Older people may locate increasingly in age-segregated housing in run-down sections of large cities, forming "ghettos of the old". Housing shortages may pit the poor young against the impoverished old, the US experts believe.

The Australian picture is dark, too. Older workers, forced to retire earlier to allow younger workers to find employment, will be hard pressed to maintain their homes. The increased number of people over 75 may swell institutions just at a time when resistance to increased taxes is expected to be very high.

In Egypt, increased numbers by the year 2000 will not give the elderly a priority over the young. No gain is expected in supportive services. The plight of an older incapacitated person in the year 2000 will be desperate. Inflation is expected to continue to raise building costs, and may prohibit the construction of new institutional facilities.

Experts in the UK see a trend toward the dissolution of the family and increasing diminution of support for the elderly. Lack of community support will further weaken the ability of families to care for their older relatives.

Poland expects no changes for the worse or the better.

Recommendations

Almost all the international experts view the future housing problems of the elderly with alarm. Yet, few nations have specific policies or programs to deal with the coming difficulties. The family is seen as the best resource for the elderly. All countries, particularly the less developed ones, view "the preservation of the family", in the words of an expert from Kenya, as a necessity for the elders. Tax relief for families that care for their elderly relatives is a common proposal by the experts.

Australia advances the idea of "inflation-proof" savings accounts to facilitate the buying of homes. The Indian experts suggest that corporations and government agencies be encouraged to promote home ownership.

Experts from the UK suggest that the government provide grants for modifications necessary to allow an aged home-owner to remain in his accustomed housing. An Australian expert suggests that the government fund improvements and then recover the costs from the older person's estate after death.

Israeli and British experts stress that coordination of agencies serving the elderly is important in maintaining independence of the elderly and ensuring that they receive full service, especially in view of trends away from inter-generational households.

Several experts recommend conversion of unused commercial or school buildings to residences for the elderly.

Experts of Sweden and Japan question the tradition of single-family homes. They advise more building of multi-family units for flexibility in accommodating the elderly and for advantageous management of initial and long-term expenses. Small housing units are suggested by the Italian experts. Prizes are proposed to encourage architectural designs both for the elderly and for multi-generational families.

French experts advise a late-life shift toward housing more suitable for old age. An older person would, at about age 60, find new housing, perhaps an apartment, that would be comfortable, agreeable, and compatible with restricted means and mobility, and move before serious disabilities set in.

Experts from Japan advise the development of a system to tap home-equity without displacing an older individual. This would allow savings accumulated in the form of equity to serve as income during the person's life-time and avoid forced sale in order to obtain funds. The Japanese experts also suggest housing loans for two-generation families living together, and the provision of rented apartments specially equipped for the elderly and built with government support. In the United States, until high interest rates appeared, a movement for "reverse annuity mortgages" was gaining converts. Such a mortgage provides the home-owner with a regular cash payment based on equity in the house; upon the home-owner's death, the mortgage-holder may pay the estate any remaining equity and take possession of the house.

The Nigerian experts consider that family planning leads to better support for the elderly in housing and other needs. A better-planned family produces members who are more socially responsible, and hence more likely to care for their elderly. The experts emphasize that family planning, and other measures supportive of the elderly (such as allowances), should be adapted to Nigerian culture and implemented so as to promote family independence. Nigeria cannot afford a pattern seen in some industrialized nations, where reliance on welfare programs for two or three generations corrodes family responsibility.

Chapter 3
PROVISION OF SERVICES

Order of priority given to "Health services and social services":

1	W GERMANY	ISRAEL	NIGERIA	
2	EGYPT	KENYA	SWEDEN	
3	ITALY			
4	BRAZIL	INDIA	POLAND	UK
5	AUSTRALIA	USA		
6	PHILIPPINES			
7	JAPAN			
8				
9	FRANCE			

The main problems today

Overview

The US experts strike a theme when they cite the phrase "alternatives to institutionalization". The phrase refers to community-based and home services. The US should think of institutions as "alternatives", say the experts.

Some champions of the elderly would argue that care of the chronically ill occurs primarily in the home with assistance of family members, neighbors, friends, and others who come together as an informal support network.

This is not to say that professionals in health and social care serve in minor roles. Clearly, they play major roles in the formal delivery of services, as do the institutions of the hospital and nursing home. However, a balanced view would accord the informal elements their rightful place in public policy considerations concerning the substance, financing, and organization of assistance to individuals in need.

Moreover, it is impossible in many instances to distinguish between health and social factors as influences on an individual's ability to maintain independence. French law implicitly recognizes this. While there may be organizational, historical, and financial reasons for the separation of health and social services, the provision of one without the other may be counter-productive or ineffective. Consequently, an ideal system delivers both.

In more developed nations, with high concentrations of professional manpower in institutions like the hospital, resources tend to be allocated more to health services than to social services, and more to acute care than to chronic care. One result is a tendency to ignore or minimize chronic care needs. Indeed, a vivid example is furnished by the medical dramas of US television, which are overwhelmingly dramas of acute illness; chronic care receives a relatively small share of public attention.

The goal of assisting a disabled individual to make adaptations and to preserve lifestyle may lack the immediate glamor of heroic efforts in acute care, but it may be equally important. The key types of assistance for the chronically ill person may take the mundane form of chore services (someone comes into the dwelling to clean, cook, and make repairs for safety and health purposes), shopping services, friendly visiting (to counter loneliness and monitor someone who may need help), and simple nursing (to change dressings and give assistance in bathing, toileting, and taking medications, in following an exercise regimen, or in using equipment).

With a spectrum of supports by the informal network and by organizations providing medical, nursing, counseling, home-health, home-maker, meals-on-wheels, friendly visiting, and other services, an elderly patient may progress through a growing burden of chronic illness – and remain at home. Senior centers, day-care centers, and other community-based services may contribute to the goal of maintaining the individual's desired living arrangements and participation in society for the longest feasible duration.

Achievement of this goal may depend also on appropriate housing. For example, consider the individual living alone in a detached house better suited to the large family of his or her earlier years. Such a person may be at more risk of mental and physical deterioration than his or her counterpart in an apartment house containing communal dining facilities and served by health and social care-givers. Such living arrangements are scarce.

For some individuals, progressive deterioration may make it necessary to live in a nursing home in which skilled nurses, therapists, and other professional care-givers are on hand. Consequently, in an ideal system of chronic care, a wide spectrum of services should be tailored to diverse and changing needs. Institutionalization may be essential to survival. Unfortunately, in many areas, the principal chronic care institution, the nursing home, is poorly developed as a site of professional care. It is isolated from centers of research and academic training. Physicians may visit irregularly. Poor working conditions may contribute to high rates of staff turnover. Scandalous conditions have been linked far more often with for-profit than other auspices.

A vocabulary for chronic care and the organized and informal delivery of services in a variety of settings is being developed in response to awareness of a growing elderly population. For want of better terms, "nursing home" stands for a wide variety of institutions, some offering little more than custodial service while others may approximate rehabilitation hospitals. "Community-based and home services" may be unclear to the public.

This chapter covers the breadth of formal chronic care services – health and social, and home, community, and institutional. Although some introductory reference is made, the subject of informal networks is reserved primarily for discussion in the chapters dealing with supports by family and community.

Institutional services

Comprehensive systems of geriatric services, as described above, are rare. In most countries that are relatively well endowed with medical and social services for the population in general, the comprehensive delivery of services to the elderly appears to have a low priority. In the less developed countries, basic structures of health and social services are lacking for everyone.

Institutional care of the elderly is almost non-existent in the less developed countries, In Kenya, experts report a lack of geriatric services, a complete absence of geriatric beds in hospitals, and no liaison between hospital and community-based services. Nigeria has only a few old people's homes, typically poorly run. Egypt has only 34 registered homes and a scant 20 geriatric beds.

Hospitals around the world are keyed, typically, to acute care, for which technologically elaborate procedures are necessary. The chronic care needs of the elderly tend to be poorly funded, and the institutions that serve them have severe staffing shortages. Rehabilitation is rarely offered. According to UK, US, and Swedish experts, doctors and nurses usually are unfamiliar with geriatrics, and tend to turn away from the elderly in frustration and even with hostility.

Institutions for the elderly tend to become "storage" facilities, many experts report. US experts cite scandals and abuses in nursing homes for the elderly, especially in for-profit facilities, where costs are said to be exorbitant and care-givers unmotivated and ill-trained to meet nursing and rehabilitation needs. Staff turnover rates are high, and repetitive training becomes necessary. As the major payers for services, federal and state governments tend to over-regulate the facilities in an attempt to secure adequate care. But the reimbursement rates tend to be protested by the owners as too low. Except for some voluntary or church-related nursing homes, the facilities tend to be isolated from the community. Total US annual spending for nursing home care exceeds $22 billion annually, half by government.

In France, good medical care is available in hospitals for the older person who requires a stay of less than 6 months. But chronic care for a longer period, and assistance with such problems as incontinence, are difficult to obtain. Many chronic care facilities are antiquated.

Community services

Few countries offer formal programs of community-based and home services. These are services that are directed toward maintaining an individual in his or her own home, and assisting families and other informal care-givers to keep an aged relative with them. These services may be given by health and social service professionals or trained lay persons, in organized programs sponsored by local government and voluntary groups. In the US, a few for-profit businesses may provide home care.

By and large, there is little public awareness of the value of such services. They tend to be placed in competition for funds with institutions – and this almost invariably is disadvantageous. On the assumption that the care they provide would be resumed by the family, these programs are likely to be the first to lose official funding.

Staffing appears to be a major problem. As the Italian response to the Sandoz Institute survey puts it, "skilled, conscientious, and efficient personnel are needed, but often 'mercenary' workers are hired, although they lack skills and motivation." In Sweden, community and home services are not available on weekends or evenings; their staffs are largely women of little education who work part-time and have their own families to attend.

Poland has a comprehensively designed system. Social help for the old and infirm is guaranteed in the Constitution. Therapy and medicines are provided free in clinics, sanatoria, and hospitals. Regional physicians, municipal dispensaries, and village health centers give medical care. The physicians are encouraged to work with teams consisting of a visiting nurse, a social assistant, and a social worker. In fact, serious problems compromise the design. For example, hospitalization is sometimes over-extended to avoid returning an older patient to poor housing.

Egypt, whose problems appear typical of a less developed country, has few services. Government officials seem convinced that the elderly are few in number and their problems are not urgent. Kenyan experts find the misconception endemic.

According to experts in Australia, the UK, Japan, West Germany, France, and the US, scarce community services are often inappropriately linked with institutional health and social services, themselves in short supply.

Policies and programs today

Institutional services

Inadequacies in beds, manpower, linkages with community and home services in health and social care, and funding are recognized throughout the surveyed countries. Some government and private actions to ameliorate these problems are reported, but the breadth and vigor of actions and plans vary considerably.

India, Kenya, Nigeria, Brazil, the Philippines, Poland, and Egypt report few, if any, policies and programs. India, for example, notes that hardly 1% of the elderly in need have access to geriatric hospitals, nursing homes, and day-care centers; there are no specific policies and programs to change the situation, the experts say. In Egypt, which has only token facilities for the elderly, the government is organizing a Society for Care of Senior Citizens to arouse interest in institutional services. The Kenyan experts, having noted a total absence of geriatric beds in their country, answer "nil" when asked what policies and programs are in effect.

Indigenous approaches to providing services deserve careful consideration, say the Nigerians. They note the Aiyetero community development scheme – thirty years ago, under a religious leader, a few hundred individuals established themselves on an island and developed a self-contained fishing and agricultural community. Cradle-to-grave needs are met on a cooperative basis.

In more developed countries, publicly- and privately-supported programs of institutional care are likely to be in various stages of development, but are nowhere near a level of comprehensiveness and quality the experts would like. Plans for reorganizing health or social systems of care to fit the needs of the elderly have been officially developed or introduced recently in several countries, notably in France, UK, Italy, Israel, West Germany, and Sweden.

The US experts note the existence of Medicare, far more directed at acute-care than chronic-care institutional services; Medicaid, a federally-aided state program for the poor that supports long-term care in nursing homes; and health maintenance organizations (HMOs), in which the services of physicians and hospitals are covered by capitation. Some HMOs have federal aid in starting up. In competition with solo, fee-for-service medicine, HMOs are wary of accepting high risk individuals or including nursing-home benefits.

Both Italy and France, say their experts, are having difficulty in implementing effective programs. According to the French, government policy is unrealistic and unsatisfactory. Measures taken under a reform law have not produced enough service capacity, funding, and staffing. A policy seeking to humanize institutions has gone awry in bureaucratic hands, producing standardization that fails to meet diverse needs of the elderly. Homes for the aged have been divided into those with nursing services and those without, preventing facilities from adapting to changing needs of residents.

Massive de-hospitalization of patients whose placement was prompted by social needs is called for under an Italian reform plan. The plan aims at promoting organized home care, specialized nursing, day hospitals, and the assignment of geriatricians to medical teams and rehabilitation experts to public dispensaries. However, the Italian experts say the plan, authorized by a 1978 law, has not gone beyond the preparatory stage and elements are still under discussion.

In the UK, a 1974 reorganization of the National Health Service was aimed at facilitating cooperation with local authorities that provide social services. However, because of economic hard times for the nation, the government's top priority is reduced spending and new projects have been halted. Recommended norms for geriatric beds (10 per 1,000 persons over age 65) and for places in residential homes (25 per 1,000) are considered inadequate and, even so, are not met in many areas. Hospitals are pressed to return patients whenever possible to their own homes. Government policy encourages community-based care and the conversion of residential homes to nursing homes.

Expansion of institutions and personnel serving the elderly is under way in West Germany and Sweden. The Swedish expansion is limited by economic conditions and competing claims on resources by advocates of acute-care services. Sweden, Australia, and Japan report programs of research and training in geriatrics.

In Israel, plans are being developed for a continuum of care covering the elderly in all stages of dependence. Reform of nursing homes is contemplated, including de-commercialization of the industry (45% of nursing homes are proprietary), elimination of small, poor quality units, and a new method of financing services.

Japan is trying to lay a foundation for a nursing-home system interlocked with the community, privately run, financed in some collective fashion, and staffed with trained professionals, including physicians. News media accounts have made the inadequacy of medical service in old people's homes clearer to the public.

The Philippines have a policy oriented away from institutionalization, except as a last resort.

The US experts cite a variety of public and private programs in support of long-term care, but lament that these do not add up to a whole system with coordinated funding, manpower supply, and quality assurance. The programs cited predominantly fall within the health services.

Need for geriatric practitioners is often noted by the experts. Lack of clear planning and policy, and implementation hamstrung by economic conditions, are also noted in several lands.

Community and home services

France, US, Australia, West Germany, Poland, and the UK have policies or programs that foster community-based or home services. Israel, while lacking a specific policy, nevertheless tries to provide home services.

The US and Australia have some successful demonstrations and established projects, but the concept of integrated community services is spreading only slowly.

Under federal funding, the US is testing a "channeling agency" concept, keyed to comprehensive assessment and referral for health, social, and other services. Nine "long-term care gerontology centers" have been established to be model systems of service, training, and research, uniting community and academic organizations; each center receives $400,000 in federal money for core activities, seeks additional private funding, and earns payment for governmental programs for an augmented list of standard benefits. The federal Veterans Administration also operates geriatrics research and training centers at its university-affiliated hospitals.

France has special community programs in 900 sectors of the country. Among the services provided are home helps, home meal services, laundry, and similar assistance. French experts say that more needs to be done to develop the quality and the quantity of these services.

Sweden has established "service houses" with about 100 apartments in each building. Each small apartment has one room, a pantry, and a bathroom. The pensioner occupants share meals in a communal dining room. Nurses and occupational therapists are on site full-time, and doctors visit the service houses each week. Sweden offers hospital-based patrols to aid the home-bound elderly and to search for older people in need of help.

Several countries are relying on recreational and other lay organizations to provide infomation or services to the elderly. In Egypt, a TV program entitled "The spring of life" carries messages to the elderly on health care and other needs. In Japan, seven million older persons, about half the elderly population, belong to old people's clubs. These recreational clubs disseminate educational messages designed for the elderly.

A ten-year policy in favor of community care in the UK has helped to keep many older people out of institutions. Recent experiments to assist the isolated elderly include boarding them in foster-care homes and the development of group homes (where three or four older people share a house, expenses, and chores).

The year 2000

The outlook in many countries is for larger populations of elderly persons, with the most rapid expansion at ages above 80. Costs of care will be up, not only because more people will be at ages where dependency rates are high due to illness, especially senile dementia, but also because of the expense of better trained manpower and technological advances.

Competition for public resources, say the Americans, will produce more ambulatory care and less hospitalization. Sensitivity to costs, however, may encourage insensitivity to quality of care for the elderly: institutions for long-term care may become warehouses. Moreover, the Americans expect that the issue of euthanasia for the most feeble, institutionalized elderly may be raised.

The UK experts are concerned about growing bureaucratic formalism, which may deaden the vitality and imagination needed in institutions serving the elderly. They expect that, if the country allocates more resources to the elderly, it will be at the expense of other sectors.

The West Germans foresee a need for more institutions to handle the increase in the over-70 population. Preparations for this eventuality must include manpower training. The Israelis, foreseeing a 60% increase in the population aged 75 and older, believe the demand for care may be met by 6,200 new long-term care beds, or a smaller number in combination with non-institutional services. The Israelis alone note that the future elderly population will have an even greater excess of women over men; these women probably will be more at risk of institutionalization, because they will have no families to turn to.

The Italians hope that better preventive measures and treatment will help to maintain high levels of health and independence for the elderly, thus minimizing need for institutions. But they do not think that the nation's social welfare system will be well organized.

The Australians foresee technological innovations that will raise the costs of care, and taxpayer resistance to meeting capital and operating costs. As a result, as service demands increase, the country may turn increasingly to the proprietary sector to meet them.

In some countries, the dissolution of rural communities at the same time that urban communities are yet to mature will have serious implications for the elderly of 2000. The experts believe that the existence or creation of sound local communities is the basis for systems of support for the dependent elderly. The Japanese experts, like the Australians, foresee proprietarization of residential and other services.

In Egypt, average life expectancy at birth will increase to 60.7 years from 54.8 today, the elderly population will enlarge, and its problems will be aggravated. Migration of young people to other countries, and to the cities from the countryside, housing problems, changes in family and economic patterns – all will conspire to make institutional care an urgent need. Yet, institutions will not be improved, working conditions will be poor, and the number of trained personnel will be inadequate, the Egyptians say.

Worsening situations for the elderly are seen in Nigeria and Brazil. In Kenya, traditional care will disappear and institutional services will not be in existence. As the concept of the extended family dies, most sick elderly persons will be stranded without care.

Sweden and Poland expect demand for institutional services to go up. The Poles see intensified shortages of beds and manpower.

Recommendations

A. Systems

A comprehensive geriatric care system should have the following elements, drawn from the experts' responses as a whole:

1. Professional staffing (doctors, nurses, paramedical personnel, social workers, mental health workers) by individuals with a back-

ground in gerontology as well as practical training in geriatric concepts and procedures. This requirement implies education and training adapted to the needs of delivering geriatric care. In-service training should be available for aides and volunteer workers.

2. Coordination of institutionally-based and community-based health-care organizations so they are mutually supportive and provide a seamless progression of services as a patient's needs intensify. This requirement implies consultation and communication across specialties and organizational affiliations.

3. Coordination of housing, health services, and social services so they, too, are mutually supportive in meeting the individual's changing needs.

4. Mechanisms of financing services, without distorting the planning and delivery of services appropriate to the individual's needs. The mechanisms may be national health insurance, tax-supported social services, subsidized housing, and private arrangements.

5. A fair balance of resources between acute and chronic care. In effect, this means reducing the great emphasis on acute care and making room for chronic care. Specifically, practitioners would be oriented toward rehabilitation.

6. Development of geriatric evaluation facilities such that abilities to carry out normal functions are gauged, and comprehensive needs of patients and families are assessed and planned for, including special living arrangements, individual and family counseling, rehabilitation, and nursing.

7. Biomedical and psychosocial research, research on the delivery of services, and research on quality-of-life issues, so that a sound scientific base for practice is assured.

8. Versatility of health-care and residential facilities to permit a variety of uses, depending on the changing needs of patients.

9. Establishment of credentials for practitioners and accreditation of institutions and agencies, to ensure quality of service.

10. Strategies for controlling costs and promoting the most cost effective services.

11. Strategies for case-finding and screening.

12. Patient and family education in good geriatric care.

Fragmentation and an incomplete spectrum of services appear

to be general concerns of experts in most countries. And these concerns merge with an appreciation of resource limitations. The experts' statements appear to carry an inner voice, most evident in the Italian call for efficiency and in the American call for rationing of health services. Reverberations are heard in a West German suggestion to use volunteers (especially young pensioners encouraged by tax breaks or money) in an effort to reduce costs, in an Israeli suggestion of a moratorium on hospital construction to free funds for social and health support systems, and in an Australian recommendation for encouragement of less costly forms of care and a discouragement of unbridled growth in institutional services.

Cost restraint, re-allocation, planning, and coordination are recurrent themes in the responses from more developed countries. Perhaps for these countries, a permissible summary view is that the evolution of care systems is out of step with population dynamics, and the main recommendations for reform add up to this message to policy-makers:

Complete your country's approach to health and social services by giving priorities to chronic care, with due attention to the simultaneous need for planning, management, and science.

B. Manpower and education

In both less developed and more developed countries, a general priority is for training more geriatrically-oriented professional, paraprofessional, and volunteer workers. Emphasis is placed on training them to work as inter-disciplinary teams, and to be familiar with preventive geriatrics and the possibilities of services in a wide variety of settings, including the home, day hospital, sheltered housing, day-care center, hospital, and nursing home. Experts in several countries call for higher salaries and qualifications, and better working conditions, to bring better personnel into chronic care.

The training of physicians in geriatrics is recommended specifically by the US, West German, Italian, Egyptian, and Polish experts. In the US, which has no formal geriatrics medical specialty, major changes in medical education have been proposed to incorporate geriatrics into the training of new physicians and the continuing education of established physicians. The concept of a "teaching nursing home", as a counterpart of the teaching hospital, has been advocated. In addition, geriatric specialists should be developed as teachers, clinical investigators, consultants, and primary care-givers or managers for cases beyond the scope of primary physicians.

In the UK, the call is for better training of social workers and well-trained professionals to manage facilities. The West Germans propose that health and social service professionals receive gerontologic and geriatric training. Along with the Australians, the West Germans emphasize psychogeriatric training to handle mental problems of the elderly.

The training of geriatric nurse-practitioners and other non-physician care givers is a US recommendation, partly as a means of economy. Recommendations for the training of nurses and paramedical personnel also are made by experts in Sweden, Italy, and Egypt. Polish experts want visiting nurses to be trained as the main coordinators of comprehensive home care.

The Japanese experts are not alone in calling for trained volunteers. Brazil, Egypt, Australia, West Germany, and the US are explicit on the subject. However, the Japanese experts express the most far-ranging approach: beginning with primary education and continuing through college and into middle age, everyone should be oriented toward organized voluntarism in support of health, social, and other services for the elderly. Public service jobs for assisting the elderly should be created locally, the Japanese experts say. The organization of elderly people themselves for such roles is considered by the West German experts.

A model program of organized volunteer help for chronically ill patients and their families exists in the UK, begun by Valerie Eaton Griffith; the British Chest, Heart, and Stroke Association coordinates groups in 39 districts. Their small staffs train volunteers to visit patients regularly in their homes, and assist them to regain lost speech and to ward off depression and loneliness. Each group sponsors a weekly recreational club and other social events for stroke patients. Transportation is provided. Each patient has an opportunity to develop personal rapport with a volunteer at a time when the family may be sorely distressed.

C. Facilities

The traditional institutions serving the chronically ill, such as hospitals and nursing homes, should be augmented by non-residential facilities, experts from a number of countries suggest. In the day hospital and day-care center, patients transported from their homes by specially equipped van, family car, or other means are given rehabilitation. By providing care during regular working hours, these facilities assist the working family to maintain an aged relative at home. The home-health agency (which can be hospital-based) sends nurses, therapists, and aides into the home for patients unable to leave.

The US experts call for measures to induce and assist health-care leaders in integrating services based on traditional and new kinds of facilities. They also propose that housing arrangements be developed in a way that facilitates the delivery of health and social services within the dwelling. The French experts propose that living arrangements for the elderly – including sheltered housing and nursing homes – provide for all the varieties of assistance they may need, including basic medical care. In addition, quality of daily life must be assured: nutritious meals, physical comfort, common rooms, television and telephone, and accessibility to and from the outside world. In the Swedish view, institutions should strive to support the patient's normal style of life.

D. Integrated services

The Polish experts are among those in several lands who espouse a variety of facilities to meet changing needs of the individual. This variety must be accompanied by methods of placing the patient in the institution that best serves his or her needs: from general hospital to home for the retired.

Many experts recommend development of geriatric evaluation units, multi-disciplinary appraisals as a prerequisite to admission to an institution, and better methods of needs assessment. The US experts emphasize assessment of functional abilities as a key to planning care. Further, they recommend that payment for services be tied to results, or outcome.

The Israelis would grant priority to developing social and health support systems in the community. The West Germans would key expansion of institutional services to integrated health and social planning, weighted toward rehabilitation and nursing.

E. Central, local, and individual control

Australian, Nigerian, and UK experts are wary of too much central government control. They call for more local authority over the management of services. The Australians would localize much of the financing of services, reinforcing local control; the national government's role would be limited to equalizing the capacities of local communities. Flexibility would be maintained through block funding of institutional and community care; those communities needing services would have access to the grantors in stating their wants.

Room for individual initiative is sought by experts from several countries, including France, Australia, and the US. The Australians propose greater reliance on the market-place by providing the elderly infirm with sufficient income or vouchers to arrange for commercial services. The US experts, while wary of proprietary services, prefer strategies with a mixture of market-place and government programs.

F. Formal and informal services

Many of the experts are concerned about relationships between professional and official organized services, and those provided informally by family, neighbors, and friends. The experts offer no well-defined mechanisms for structuring the relationships, but they unanimously consider both kinds of service providers to be essential to the elderly.

Without informal services, many elders would not be assisted at all. Great loads would be placed on already over-burdened professional facilities and organizations, and could be met only at enormous social expense.

Experts in a wide range of countries propose ways of helping families to help their elders. One major approach is to provide those professional and volunteer services that bring problems within manageable proportions for the informal care-givers. This category would include services at home or during the day in health and social facilities, such as hospitals and senior centers. The home services would be provided by professionals, especially nurses and physical therapists, as well as lesser-skilled personnel, such as home-health aides and home-makers.

Another major approach is to subsidize the true or surrogate family (e.g., foster home) in maintaining the elder. The US experts speak of "family incentives", the Indians of "subsidies to poor families", and the British of "financial support to kith and kin". The Australians would like to set up pilot projects to evaluate "boarding out" of older people who have no supporting families to turn to. The Italians suggest that the State remunerate private individuals and organizations willing to help the dependent elderly.

The breadth of the above recommendations appears warranted by the scope of needs encountered in evolving societies. As the US experts put it, "What is needed is a total re-conceptualization and re-organization of the total health and welfare system."

Chapter 4
PAYMENT FOR SERVICES

Overview

This chapter departs from the general plan of exposition by omitting a section on "Policies and programs today", as these are closely intertwined with "The main problems today" affecting payment for services.

The problems of payments must be viewed with an eye to many of the other issues considered in the Sandoz Institute survey. Income in retirement, family and community support, and volunteer activities, as well as provision of services, bear upon costs and ability to pay.

Payment for services can be approached from several angles, principally: cost of services to the client or patient; revenues available to the service organization from reimbursement, direct charges, philanthropy, and government subsidy; and what society as a whole pays, in taxes and privately, as a percentage of gross national product.

At probably no other single point do the problems of a growing elderly population come into conflict more clearly with other social priorities than in the context of payment for health and social services.

The amount of payment for these services by retirees has obvious implications for their standard of living. Service charges may constrict already tight budgets for food, clothing, shelter, and other essentials, possibly endangering the very independence the services may aim to preserve. Moreover, social status, mental and physical well-being, and self image may be undermined by threats to, or actual declines in, living standards for those in or near poverty.

Services may be provided without direct charge to the individual, thus protecting living standard. They may be provided at a nominal charge or at a charge geared to income level through a means test, thus splitting the cost between beneficiary and third-party payers, including government. In many countries, payment appears to be more generous if the service is labeled as a health service. In the realm of long-term care, which involves costs of room and board, cleaning and other custodial or hotel services, recreational services, nursing, rehabilitation, speech and other therapies, and physicians' services, the definition of costs is complex and arbitrary. A change in categorization of patient (as needing skilled or lesser nursing, as likely to recover with active therapy or not, as being poor or not), or whether the service is a health or other service, may affect who is obligated to pay and how much of the cost is recognized for third-party payment.

Payment may be from public and private pools, such as tax revenues or insurance. Burdens on the tax system may add to pressure for tax reform and increase inter-generational conflict. As a matter of conserving these funds, public policy-makers may be attracted to means testing, larger deductibles and cost sharing, tighter eligibility requirements, and longer lists of excluded services. In the United States, Medicare over the years has been covering less and less of personal health expenditures for the elderly; it now covers 40% or less. Shifting more expense to the beneficiary may pose threats to living standard, including health status, and create tensions within the family and community.

Payment problems are politically charged issues. The creation of benefits paid by a governmental program may establish constituencies of beneficiaries and providers of service. Their special interest in shaping or preventing legislative and regulatory changes is intensified in periods of retrenchment. An incomplete set of service benefits for the elderly may remain incomplete in the competition for funds, particularly by providers of current benefits. Prospects of expanding long-term care services are particularly at risk.

The design of insurance influences costs, quality, and accessibility of care. In so far as insurance improves the individual's ability to pay or be paid for, costs or charges will increase in the absence of controls on providers of care. Often the need for cost curbs is obvious, but a scientific basis is lacking for designing them with the least upset to professionally sound courses of patient or client management. In Italy, measures are being taken to control drug costs and shorten hospital stays, but they are not based on objective research. Even where providers are employed by government, costs may rise despite attempts at austerity. Difficulties in constructing controls that are effective and perceived to be fair to beneficiary and provider seem to be never ending.

The main problems today

Stagnating economies, inflation generally and in health services especially, lack of third-party coverage for long-term care for the non-poor, under-financing and fragmented financing of services, and inadequate policy-making appear to be major problems in paying for services.

MORE DEVELOPED COUNTRIES

Basic problems of the more developed countries seem to be exemplified by West Germany. In a stagnating economy, the massive social insurance system – including sickness, pension, disability, and unemployent benefits – is under stress. Unemployment benefit demands go up while the system's ability to pay goes down: there is shrinkage in the earnings on which taxes are based. Citizens are pushed to the limits of their abilities to pay taxes in general, the West German experts say.

Meanwhile, costs of health and social services are rising, partly as a result of inflation, the increasing numbers of elderly persons, and more expensive manpower and technology in health care. The elderly are hurt financially. Out-of-pocket payments for health services go up. The expenses of residence in an old-age or nursing home, which are not covered by social insurance or private insurance, gut pensions and force the elderly to seek social aid or support from their children. Psychological effects are adverse. Moreover, the state of the economy precludes improvements in West German pension and service benefits.

Long-term care

While social insurance falls short of maintaining classic protections, it is unable to expand. Systematizing long-term care and its funding appears to be even further beyond reach while needs for individual relief continue to grow. In various countries, middle-income people are hard hit by direct nursing-home expenses. In the US, expenditures for nursing-home care have been rising faster than inflation in general and faster than hospital expenditures. Long-term care costs in West Germany and Australia are more than the individual can handle. Shopping for an affordable private nursing home in Australia leads many individuals into substandard places.

In the US, no private insurance coverage exists for these services. A federal-state program, Medicaid, covers nursing-home expenses of the poor in varying degree. Middle-income individuals must become poor before eligibility for Medicaid is granted. In many cases, the elderly private payer becomes impoverished after a period in a nursing home as a private patient. Whether the individual remains there or is re-located depends on the facility's policy of accepting Medicaid reimbursement.

Categorical conflicts

In general, payment for health services is favored over social services. The public in Sweden supports a priority to health-care funding, for example. In economic hard times, social services tend to lose ground first. Within the health-care sphere, acute care services tend to hold their ground more than long-term care services, and institutional services tend to fare better than new community-based and home services. One result is that an already patchwork system may deteriorate, with severe impact on the vulnerable elderly population.

"There is a constant effort to make things look as though we are doing something, even when we are not," comments an American expert. In large measure, he continues, current problems in financing are due to tight categorical allocations. Eligibility varies from program to program, and incorrect placement in a program is often a result of an individual's being eligible for that program, rather than the ineptitude of administrators.

Different financing roots play a part in complicating access to services. In the UK, where both health and social services are considered under-financed, service boundaries are confusing to the public. For example, hospital care is free, while community services are means-tested and carry an aura of charity: social-services administrators seem to take a punitive attitude toward applicants, the UK commentators say.

Dodging responsibility

Hospital and community (local authority) institutions in the UK resist collaboration. Services are poorly deployed. Passing the buck between health and social-service authorities is reported to be common in Italy. Under these conditions, elderly persons and their families are perplexed about their rights and opportunities and, in Australia, may resort to private insurance even though entitled to free care as pensioners for certain services. In the US, many elderly persons buy private insurance to fill in "gaps" in the Medicare program; many of these policies are considered to be excessively expensive for the benefits provided.

In Israel, multiple funding sources and jurisdictions leave some people with no coverage at all and some kinds of services uncovered, such as dental care. While sick funds provide assured financing for acute care in hospitals and for physicians' services, the ministry of welfare pays a share of home-health, meals-on-wheels, and other home services only if a local share is raised. Otherwise, there is no obligation to provide the services. Meanwhile, sick funds are not responsible for extended nursing care. The Israeli experts see a great need for systematization by establishing mandatory national health insurance, priorities for developing social support services, and funding mechanisms for these services. Israel may be unique among governments by having a law committing itself in principle to the design of a long-term care system. A commission is studying the incorporation of insurance premiums for long-term care coverage as part of a social security system.

Japan has an unusual problem, typical of the difficulties that can develop out of piecemeal planning for medical insurance. In Japanese hospitals, the experts report, there are extra fees for attendants who bathe and feed severely ill patients. These extra costs can add up to a heavy financial burden, and the experts believe that they should be covered as part of basic medical care.

Age discrimination by cost control

To resolve problems arising when benefit expenses exceed income into an insurance program, administrators may place payment limits on amount or kind of service. The limits may work against medical or other care needs of the patient. The French experts give the example of a hemiplegic patient who requires prolonged rehabilitation after surgery. An arbitrary limit on length of covered hospital stay for active treatment may force the patient's transfer into a payment category that does not cover the needed care. To continue proper treatment, the patient has to make large out-of-pocket payments. These work to impoverish the patient, so that after a full course of care there are no home and other resources left for independent living. The patient, often humiliated, becomes a public assistance recipient.

Attempts by central government to economize may shift obligations to municipalities. The step may be justified as decentralization. Yet, the French point out, the burden may be harder for some localities to meet than for others. Those with less industry and more emigration of young adults may find themselves contending with a growing proportion of elderly persons and a dwindling tax base, the French experts point out. The elderly in such places may lose supportive services.

Payments may be stringent for home services, and limits may be placed by maximum number of hours per day, subsidized according to the patient's income. At the same time, costly medical techniques and over-specialization boost hospital costs, which the public more willingly pays.

Governmental austerity may fall unevenly on the elderly. While spending for services may be reduced, extravagant pensions may be awarded to some individuals. Increasingly, people are becoming accustomed to being claimants and thus are less likely to forego benefits because the steps needed to qualify for them are unpleasant.

Under-financing of services is cited by experts in several countries. Services are free in Poland but the quality and availability are limited. Italian experts state that 5.9% of the nation's gross national product goes for health care, but this is inadequate for effective services. As a minimum, a large increase in social insurance – of the order of 10–20% – would be needed to provide an adequate funding base for services to the aged.

Sweden spends 32% of gross national product for social welfare, including 9% for health care. The tax burden confines the country's ability to maintain the services at their current level. Indeed, public resentment of taxes is producing cries for direct fees.

LESS DEVELOPED COUNTRIES

In the less developed countries, health and social services are under-financed, facilities and manpower are lacking, and large segments of the elderly population are too poor to pay for services, or are otherwise excluded from them. The elderly poor in India are entitled to free health services, which, the experts note, are ineffective and inadequate. Treatment for chronic illness is not available in institutions because of bed shortages. Traditional healing services are available.

In Nigeria, where about 1.8% of the national budget is for health care and the per capita expenditure is about one US dollar per year, only 30% of the population has coverage. Insufficient funding characterizes Egypt's health services. While they are provided free in general hospitals run by the government, no special services for the elderly are available. Inadequate coverage also is the case in Brazil, and long-term care is complicated by poor coordination between government agencies responsible for health and social services. Kenya lacks basic data to identify problems in delivery of services.

Employment and insurance are clearly interwoven, with many plans being totally or partially financed by employers. This can be a sad fact of life for a retired worker in less developed as well as more developed countries. Sometimes insurance programs exclude those who have never worked, to say nothing of those too poor to obtain insurance. In the Philippines, for instance, the unemployed and the retired are not covered. In Egypt, insurance is limited in scope, and, among the elderly, available only to retired employees of major organizations or the government.

The year 2000

Experts in most countries foresee crises in the funding of services.

By the year 2000 France will have 1.5 million persons aged 80 and over; only one in four will be autonomous, and the rest will require massive institutional and community services. Claimant mentality will over-strain social services in West Germany, and more one-person households will mean higher assistance costs.

In Australia, because of taxpayer resistance, the government will reduce subsidies and narrow eligibility for benefits, thus shifting expenses to families and philanthropic organizations.

In the US, family and social networks will erode at the same time that service programs falter for lack of funds. The American experts believe the nation will have to agree on payment roles for government, private insurance, and the individual; at worst, most elderly will be exposed to personal bankruptcy in paying for services if they want anything better than "warehousing". Senile dementia will cause an exponential rise in the need for services.

In Poland, personnel shortages will grow as more families are unable or unwilling to care for the ill older person. Israel's services will be strained by the expansion of the population aged 75-plus and by inflation. Japan will have to revise present payment and provision arrangements in order to avoid difficult funding problems.

Conflict will grow among social groups in Sweden as a consequence of funding problems. "The question for Swedish health care and social security is how to offer an improved care system to the elderly within today's limited economic resources," that country's experts say.

The French foresee possible confrontations between two pressure groups: the very aged and their children approaching retirement, and the general "working" population, shrunken by earlier retirement and an increasingly later start on careers. The confrontation will be sharpened if health insurance is expanded to cover complete care for the chronically ill at home or in institutions and to reduce out-of-pocket payments. The burden on the working age population will be enlarged also because the dependency ratio will rise, assuming low birth rates and continuation of taxation for social security in such a way that low-income contributors pay proportionately more of their income than do the wealthy.

In less developed countries inadequate funding will persist, with more need, further inflation, and rising expectations, according to observers in Nigeria, the Philippines, Kenya, India, and Egypt. India sees costs rising threefold, and Egypt's experts believe government funds will be unable to meet the needs of the frail elderly.

Italy sees more State planning and less personal attention, as consequences of dramatic inflation in expenditures for the aged.

Recommendations

The experts consider a variety of strategies for paying for health and social services. Some of these appear to represent a shift of responsibility between public and private sectors, or between collective and individual arrangements. The options generally appear to be considered in the context of continuing economic austerity.

The approaches suggested from less developed countries essentially adopt basic modes of more developed countries. For example, Nigerian experts advise establishing contributory health insurance, and the Indians health and social service coverage through the work-place for retired employees and dependents. The Egyptians propose encouraging private organizations to finance health and social services, with donations on behalf of the elderly to be tax deductible. The experts in Kenya propose governmental payment for comprehensive plans of health and social services, both in rural areas and in towns.

By and large, the approaches from the more developed countries go beyond public and private financing to include methods of (a) stretching available funds – by making services more efficient and effective, by restrictions on charges of providers, by administrative economies, and by using volunteers to give services; (b) lessening the use of services – by introducing user fees, and by changes in eligibility, such as stricter medical, social, and financial criteria; and (c) by increasing the job opportunities of the elderly so they can pay directly for services or buy insurance coverage.

Some of the proposals are presented under other sections of the survey, such as optimization of human resources and employment.

The West German experts suggest that preventive medical measures in middle age would help lower costs later in life. Measures to keep older people active might lead to reduced costs of care, they say, while cost sharing by patients would emphasize personal responsibility for costs of care. After calling for rationalization of the assistance system and the creation of an insurance mechanism covering long-term care, the West German experts add this statement: "In general, all financing problems of the health and social services would be solved if it were possible to divert a large part of armaments expenditure to social action."

The absence of coverage for long-term care is recognized by the

Israeli experts. Such coverage should be part of legislatively defined entitlements to services, implemented by national health insurance. A law to accomplish this has been approved in principle. As for social services, payments should not be assumed by the public budget without careful examination. In principle, as with health services, social services should be funded at no cost to the elderly.

The Americans believe the need for services can be reduced by finding effective preventive measures and treatments for senile dementia, by finding (through experimentation) effective incentives for families to care at home for their elderly, and by encouraging prepaid medical and hospital care through health maintenance organizations, subsidized, if need be, for the elderly. Private insurance, for-profit services, earnings limits on providers, and outcome based reimbursement are suggested.

The Australian experts, recalling that the expense of a free medical and hospital care program became politically intolerable and led to the program's gutting, note that the present government is seeking to impose user fees. The experts suggest that services be provided only on the basis of defined medical, social, and/or financial need. Medical need should be defined by geriatric assessment teams. To cover the growing elderly population, additional revenue sources are required, possibly taxes on sales, lump sum retirement payments, and retirement and in-kind services.

The UK experts see no realistic alternative to government-financed health and social services for the elderly. Means testing should be abolished as counter-productive; the costs of administration may be almost as high as the "savings". The experts believe that a package of health and welfare benefits, financed by a single mechanism, should be considered. "Many crucial decisions are essentially political and depend on a consensus view of social justice," they say.

The Italian experts want to reduce waste, particularly the unnecessary granting of disability pensions. The Japanese call for a corporate annuity to help those on low state pensions, control of inflation, improved medical care, and raising the retirement age to 65. The Swedes would stretch the kroner by making services more efficient and effective.

The use of volunteers is mentioned by several countries: the Poles, for example, call for developing forms of mutual aid for old people, such as the able elderly assisting the disabled, the young helping the elderly with domestic tasks, and the elderly helping young parents by looking after their children. The Filipino experts suggest measures to give the elderly maximum opportunity to render volunteer services. The American experts envisage a corps of young and old volunteers.

All health services should be covered by health insurance, say the French experts, so that medical requirements are not distorted and locale of treatment (at home or institution) is determined by state of health and patient's wishes. The-room-and-board charge to patients for long-term stays should be identical in all institutions, so that decisions on an appropriate place can be made without regard to these "hotel" costs.

Chapter 5
OPTIMAL UTILIZATION OF HUMAN RESOURCES

The main problems today

The experts generally discuss optimal utilization in terms of professional and other trained manpower, younger volunteers, and the elderly in service to themselves and society at large in paid or volunteer capacities.

The major obstacles appear to be the under-valuing of the elderly, a corresponding depreciation of those serving them as manifested in poor pay and scarce or weak training efforts, and the absence of effective management and manpower recruitment. The healthy elderly, identified as an unused resource, have few recognized outlets for serving their communities, and lack training and organization as volunteers.

The Italian experts take a very broad approach to "optimal utilization" of human resources. They note that the economy of their country wastes human labor in such ways as the production of worthless or harmful goods, the misallocation of jobs (the young get sedentary jobs and the elderly get arduous work), and the diversion of public assistance to persons who can do without it while the needy cannot obtain emergency help because assistance personnel are lacking.

According to the UK commentators, many care-givers adopt a counter-productive approach when they give service as a matter of sufferance and induce patients to be passive and submissive. Little effort is made to draw patients and families into the process of making decisions about care, and thus opportunities are foregone to improve the plans for treatment and lifestyle adjustment.

The Nigerian commentators identify an impediment in the refusal of doctors, nurses, and government officials to collaborate with traditional healers, cultural societies, and the public in planning and providing services for the elderly.

The Poles note that there are too few social workers, and they are not well trained. Indifference to geriatric problems also is noted among physicians and nurses in several countries. The French experts point out that, since some elderly persons are hard to work with, proper motivation and organization of staff are essential. Short-ages of staff, as well as poor training in interpersonal and technical skills, are noted explicitly by experts in more developed and less developed countries – Kenya, the Philippines, Egypt, Nigeria, Brazil, as well as Australia, West Germany, US, UK, and France.

The Australians note lack of training in social gerontology and geriatrics. Professional authoritarianism inhibits initiative and co-operation among care-givers, qualities which may be as important as technical competence in achieving desired results. Rigid hierarchies imposed by licensing and funding agencies are decried by the Australian experts, because rigidity precludes innovative use of less skilled persons, such as assignment of simple nursing tasks to aides. The Australians note that voluntary services are poorly coordinated and that emphasis on for-profit nursing homes may inhibit a real caring attitude toward patients.

Indifferent orientation of health and social service personnel toward geriatrics is an American observation. Development of know-ledge of geriatrics has lagged, say the Americans. The Swedes point out that the care system for the elderly has drawn on acute care models that are inappropriate to chronic care needs.

Turning to the use of the elderly, the experts appear to agree that ignoring them as a productive social resource is a major problem. The United States only recently has started to consider seriously that adults are human capital resources to be developed through adult education, re-training, and rehabilitation. The direction of change in thinking about the elderly and other adults is away from considering these activities to be a hand-out and toward considering them to be an investment. Age prejudice in employment reflects the lack of a human capital program geared to the realities of the lifecycle, the Americans say.

Mutual aid in the home and in communities is poorly developed in Poland, Israel, and France, their experts declare. "The greatest potential (human resource) is among the elderly themselves," declare the French, "because they have the experience, will, capacity, and ideas." Efforts to encourage and apply these attributes are greatly needed. Moreover, if society encourages the elderly person to par-ticipate in productive activities while healthy, that person will have the sense of self-esteem and the will to participate in his or her own care. Without this will, the efforts of family, neighbors, and profes-sionals will very likely be in vain. According to the French, family and voluntary workers can make important contributions to the care of the elderly if given orientation, direction, and organization.

Shortages of programs for mobilizing the elderly are noted in societies as different as Israel and the Philippines. In Egypt, while inactivity is incorporated in the role society fashions for elders, they tend to receive less assistance from volunteers; the younger generation focuses increasingly on paid employment. In India, the elderly are used, but not well, by the agrarian and joint family system. Retirees tend to be idle, and employment of the elderly is discouraged generally except for menial jobs. Lack of vocational guidance for the elderly is seen in Brazil with a despairing eye, since unemployment is so rampant for all ages.

Policies and programs today

Many countries lack, or have token or unclear programs and policies for, optimal use of human resources, according to the experts.

The Swedes see progress in their care system. Organizational improvements are occurring, particularly in the use of smaller working groups of professionals with responsibility for a defined group of institutionalized patients and in the increased use of paramedical personnel. The Swedish systems of care are searching for better forms of cooperation among patients, families, and professionals. For example, the potentials and limits of geriatrics are explained, patients and families are encouraged to participate in decision-making about therapy, and provision of day care in a hospital is guaranteed if relatives assist in a plan of support.

No specific programs exist in the UK to stimulate the entry of young professionals into health and social services for the elderly. Until the recent US wave of austerity in federal funding, an emphasis on geriatrics was growing in American health-professional schools, including nursing and medicine. Geriatric and gerontological social-work programs in the US aim to improve knowledge and attitudes, the experts note.

Geriatric training for health and social service workers is improving in Poland, West Germany, Australia, and Egypt. Kenya has no training policies.

In terms of training the elderly for service, the United States government is one of the few with a program. Several countries have local or regional private programs. Old people are being enlisted in local volunteer activities in Japan through their clubs. In Israel, there is some activity by pensioners organized on the basis of former affiliation with trade unions, the civil service, universities, and the army. Attempts have been made to mobilize young groups in Israel to visit and help the elderly and to record their folk tales and life experiences. British schoolchildren are encouraged to work with or on behalf of the elderly in their communities, and several volunteer agencies provide bereavement counseling and other services of specific benefit to the elderly. Sweden is exploring increased elder participation in volunteer or philanthropic activities.

In Poland, local groups are mobilized to assist the elderly; the scope of activities varies according to local initiative and potential. The Australian elderly furnish service by volunteering, including foster grandparent programs. In the Philippines, similar programs exist. The Egyptian government is seeking ways to attract public support for local services to the elderly. India has no clear government policies and programs, though the experts note that rural communities and families have a place for the elderly as advisors.

Nigeria is building a basic health service scheme. Service networks, covering groups of 150,000 people, will each include a comprehensive health center, four primary health centers, 20 health clinics, and five mobile teams in remote areas. Except for the comprehensive center, the units are to be entirely operated by nonprofessionals, such as community health aides and assistants. Community participation and self-reliance are other features of the plan. With only 30% of today's population covered by conventional health services, Nigeria must train auxiliary health workers and strengthen collaboration with traditional healers and village health workers. The plan is to provide health care and jobs, while making efficient use of resources and correcting maldistribution of facilities.

The Year 2000

Shortages of qualified professional and paraprofessional personnel for serving the elderly in 2000 are foreseen widely as a function of growth of the aged population and demand for better care. Shortages are expected in a range of countries, such as the US, Japan, Kenya, the Philippines, Egypt, and Brazil. Most countries believe that current problems of optimizing human resources will be aggravated.

A particular worry is that reliance on government and professionals to serve the elderly will increase, largely as a result of eroding family and friendship ties. As women increase their work-force participation, family support will wane, according to the West German experts. Excessive reliance on professionals will result in part from an over-estimation of the attainability of solutions to human problems by professional and technical means.

The combination of reliance on government and professionalization is seen negatively by UK experts. They believe that professionals may find themselves distanced even further than today from their clients or patients because of their own mystiques and defensive postures. The Australians see continuing lack of inter-disciplinary cooperation.

The American experts believe the elderly will be in danger of being "warehoused" and in "public internment" as service and training costs escalate. Some elderly individuals may defer needed services because of inability to pay, but sooner or later, needing them, they will spend themselves into poverty, at which time they will qualify for government support. By then, however, deterioration will be harder to treat.

A triad of deficiencies identified by the Philippine commentators will be harmful to the elderly in various countries: shortage of qualified care-givers, lack of organized volunteers, and limited programs for utilizing the elderly productively. The Australians would add public apathy to this list.

Some optimistic notes are registered. The Israelis see a better integrated elderly population in 2000. Many more of the elderly will be better educated, speak Hebrew, understand Israeli culture, and hold professional positions. Their demands, expectations, and capacity for continued work will be higher than those of today's elderly. Mandatory retirement will be less acceptable. However, even if unemployment is relatively low for the nation, the elderly of 2000 are likely to find themselves in competition for jobs with younger workers.

The Polish experts see future retirees as being better educated and more able and willing to prevent infirmity. Consequently, demands for better trained physicians and nurses in geriatrics will increase, as well as for a complete system of social services. If people prepare better for old age, self-sufficiency may be the rule by the year 2000, the Italian experts suggest. International migration of younger workers may alter the age-group pattern, presumably stressing an Italian economy that must provide for growing numbers of elderly.

The Brazilians see a growing need for re-training older workers so they may qualify for jobs using new technology. The Indian experts see a trend toward earlier retirement, and therefore more unemployment among older workers and more idleness in retirement as life expectancy increases.

Recommendations

These parallel the dichotomy observed in the delineation of problems. On the one hand, the experts call for improved and enlarged training in geriatrics for all health professionals. On the other hand, they call for greater participation of families and individuals in care or self-care, and for greater opportunities for the elderly to continue in the work-force and express themselves through volunteer work and mutual assistance.

Experimentation in delivery of services and in work arrangements is emphasized by experts from several countries. They believe that successful experiments could be bases for permanent changes.

For example, the Americans propose experiments to develop innovative services for the elderly, as well as experiments in family incentives or supports for their care and the systematic use of public insurance, prepaid group health plans, and for-profit health services. They also propose experiments with mutual aid among the elderly using vouchers as the basis for exchange of volunteer services (a model of which is Link Opportunity, which originated in the UK). Social welfare research appeals to the Japanese. The Egyptians specifically want medical as well as social service research to be recognized as needed to meet contemporary problems. The Americans are unique among the experts in vigorously recommending research on senile dementia as part of a massive research effort to find ways of keeping individuals mentally fit.

Optimal use of human resources goes beyond a simple search for efficiency. The UK experts urge that the elderly be drawn into consultative and decision-making processes affecting health and social services. For example, they assert that any form of client participation would benefit the activities of nursing homes and home-help groups. One example of such participation would be residents' committees in nursing homes.

Several themes seem to converge on the issue of lay and professional collaboration: State paternalism and professional authoritarianism are counter-productive to optimal use of human resources; geriatric and gerontological knowledge should be disseminated among lay and professional publics; and leadership needs to be created for mobilizing the lay side of organized lay-professional cooperation.

Decentralizing government bureaucracy is espoused by the British. They say professionals and lay persons may need re-education to rely on their own judgment. The Swedes say it is important to involve families and individuals in giving care or in self-care, and to reduce governmental programs. They call for experiments in effective organization of peers and neighbors to support the elderly in their localities. For example, they would like to have pensioner associations drawn upon for friendly visitors, who might help prevent isolation and serve as forward elements of professional outreach or case-finding activities.

The West Germans, Filipinos, Egyptians, and Kenyans also manifest concern for mutual aid, self-care, and community programs. The Kenyans believe demands for primary care should be met by training elderly and other lay persons to be of assistance where professionals are in short supply.

The Egyptians insist on incorporating geriatric knowledge in medical, nursing, and social science curricula. The Brazilians want foreign technical assistance for training geriatric teams. The West Germans call for improved continuing education of professionals, including efforts to foster geriatrics as a second specialty. The Israelis and Nigerians seek expansion of geriatric training for professional and paraprofessional persons. The Israelis specify efforts to foster gerontology as a specialty within nursing, social work, and medicine.

The Polish experts advance five points that appear to summarize the multiple concerns of their counterparts in other countries. For optimizing human resources, needed measures include: raising the qualifications of practitioners in geriatrics teams; popularizing geriatrics and gerontology as part of regular education; establishing university departments of social gerontology, and schools for advanced training of social workers in geriatrics; organizing mutual aid among old people based on pensioner groups and senior citizen clubs; and preparing and disseminating health maintenance information through the mass media and adult education. A sixth point, covered only by the Poles, is the adaptation of short-term hospitals for geriatric rehabilitation.

Of all the recommendations concerning optimal use of human resources in the economy at large, one of the most fundamental is made by the Israeli experts. After noting needs for phased retirement and other means of making use of the skills and capacities of the elderly, the Israeli experts declare: "Structural changes in the economy would have to take place with priority in investing in labor rather than capital."

Phased retirement, with the elderly being shifted into less taxing jobs as required, would be only one possibility. Others include part-time jobs and specially designed jobs for the elderly. Innovations should proceed from experimentation and produce permanent reorganization of industry; for example, one company created a special department for elderly workers, where they work a shorter day at a special salary.

Another fundamental recommendation, though less concretely exemplified, concerns a life cycle perspective on productive contribution to society. Such a perspective should be presented to the young, including orientation on the need for re-training to meet conditions of later life, according to the Italian and Indian experts. The Americans would inculcate such a view in two ways: by formal and informal campaigns against age prejudice, focusing especially on employers, so that the principle "young is better" is removed from employment practices; and by developing a voluntary National Corps of Youth and Age, to foster inter-generational understanding and respect.

Community solidarity is a strong theme for the Japanese, who recommend that medical, welfare, education, and other services be associated with community facilities for the elderly. The Japanese experts would incorporate knowledge of social services into school curricula, partly to encourage careers in social services and partly to make the public aware of resources and needs. The Japanese also would use community facilities for the elderly and other organizations to help match jobs and elderly skills.

To round out the major elements of a supportive system, the Japanese would incorporate service to society as a concept and practice for students, laying a basis for volunteer activities in all of adult life. Turning to issues involved in utilizing the elderly productively for society, the Japanese appear to be searching for softening or circumventing the effects of fixed-age retirement. The lifetime employment system sponsored by companies does help retirees to find jobs, but often these are peripheral jobs unsuited to their capabilities. Corporations for the aged, subsidiaries formed by major businesses and manned by their retirees, do exist but in small number. This model effort might be expanded. Separate enterprises suited to highly educated scientific and technical personnel might be established. Inventories of jobs and retiree skills would help locate and match people to employer needs.

India needs to formulate a policy that would allow the elderly to continue in jobs until unfit to work, say the experts from that country. They also recommend development of cottage industries in rural areas to help counter-balance migration to the cities. Because workers migrate internationally, the Italians believe nations should collaborate in meeting problems that arise when the migrants become old away from their native lands. Joint programs and efforts to balance migration are suggested by the Italians.

The Filipino experts appear to be alone in characterizing reduction of institutionalization as a step to relieve demands on human resources. They propose organizing the elderly to be volunteer aides and to work in programs of national development.

Chapter 6

THE INDIVIDUAL AND THE FAMILY

Order of priority given to "Family":

1				
2	NIGERIA	POLAND		
3				
4	AUSTRALIA	FRANCE	JAPAN	SWEDEN
5	EGYPT	INDIA	KENYA	UK
6	ITALY	USA		
7	BRAZIL	ISRAEL	PHILIPPINES	
8	W GERMANY			
9				

Overview

The family is the greatest single source of support, and the center of activity, for most elderly persons. The family may be considered with regard to the elderly couple alone, or the elderly couple or person in relation to parents, children, siblings, and other relatives.

The growth of three, four, and even five-generation families under conditions of urbanization and industrialization produces unprecedented challenges and opportunities. The adaptation of families to these circumstances is poorly understood, and myths about family behavior persist from the past. Attempts to articulate the challenges and opportunities must first surmount these outmoded concepts. For example, characteristics attributed to the family in the past assumed several generations under one roof. This is true far more today than in the past, when extended families consisted not so much of children, parents, and grandparents, as of children, parents, and uncles and aunts. In the United States, only in the last 50 years has a ten-year-old child had more than a 50% chance of having two live grandparents.

Another misconception is based on confusion with the term "household". A two-generation household may be separate from, but have close ties to, a grandparental household. The separation does not necessarily indicate abandonment of the elderly by the young, but it may impede direct assistance.

Tomorrow's elderly may be as different from today's as these elderly are different from their forebears. In many countries, today's elderly have more children than their children will have, assuming continuation of relatively low birth-rates. The "baby boom" elderly will have fewer children to turn to, but more siblings. This has policy implications, in that the family of a sick elder may have no relative but aged siblings to turn to.

Another impact on family role and support derives from the longer life expectancy of women. This differential is increasing, with the result that women face more years in widowhood than ever before, possibly without support of husband's family. Other impacts concern divorce, informal cohabitational arrangements, and the ability of a younger family to share a household with elders, assuming the dwelling permits. Finally, severe chronic illness may make living with children or in their own household impossible for the elderly person or couple, and institutionalization of one spouse may make independent living impossible or complicated for the other. In some countries, middle-aged women have growing labor-force participation rates. They are no longer at home to give care to a sick elder.

To the extent that the family is unable or unwilling to support the elderly person, formal or informal assistance becomes necessary. The elderly may have to depend on community services for care the family cannot give. The cost of formal services to replace care given by the family may be enormous in the aggregate, assuming the services are available. This possibility raises the issue of the extent and type of supports that should be provided to families to permit them to continue caring for their elderly. Would payments be made unnecessarily to families that need no incentive to continue providing support? How much saving would occur through family incentives? Would payments deter institutionalization when it is appropriate? How much would be saved in institutional costs through family incentives? What would be the psychological effect of such payments?

The elderly tend to keep major family roles in rural areas of less developed countries. In urbanizing areas of those countries and in the more developed lands, the elderly play less structured roles. Little is known about family relationships in dynamic societies.

In traditional societies, the wisdom and experience of the older person are still considered pertinent to major family tasks. However, in societies undergoing relatively rapid socio-economic changes, the older person's experience tends to be discounted.

In less developed countries and Japan, old religious emphases on honoring parents still hold; by and large, caring for the elderly is seen as an important family duty. This pattern begins to break down, say experts from the Philippines and Brazil, as urbanization advances. And in more developed countries – such as Australia, Italy, the US, and the UK – older people prefer to live in their own households, but near a son or daughter. Since adult children may change residence for employment reasons, parents may be left behind. The older person is likely to have no formal role or function in the household headed by an adult child, and may end up in a very isolated and deprived condition.

Women seem to fare better than men with regard to a continued and valued role in the family, as so many of them have work patterns often of a household nature that can continue into their later years. Men, on the other hand, tend to retire, either formally or informally.

The main problems today

"Change" seems to be the key. It is occurring at a rapid rate all over the world, and the elderly are perhaps the group least able to deal with swift technological, social, and financial change.

Successful adaptation is so taken for granted that few countries have policies to bolster the family in caring for elders. A new awareness is emerging that, as the UK experts put it, "we must take care of the carers." All too often families have been divided by migration within a country or even, as is true for many old Israelis, from one country to another. In Australia, the very size of the country can isolate children and parents when they are separated geographically.

The Sandoz Institute survey shows cautious optimism that such disruption, now at its peak, will soon improve. Future generations, settled into an urbanized pattern, may not be so dramatically divided by cultural change as is the case today. According to Japanese experts, many of today's rural elders are separated from their urban children, a post-World War II occurrence. The future elderly will be lifelong urban residents.

The ability of the elderly to pay their way is considered important to the younger household. Inability to do so causes tension, say experts in countries as diverse as Brazil and the US. The US experts report that an adult's identity and self-esteem may be tied not only to work and to income, but also to a role as a consumer. All three of these roles may be impossible for an older person living on a reduced pension.

103

Older people who retain wealth are a privileged group. In Italy, they may play a major and despotic role within their families.

In most countries, the elderly add their pensions to the family income. Brazil and India are among less developed countries that have established small pensions for the elderly, so that they might make this contribution and solidify their position in the family unit. Any degree of freedom of choice added by funds contributed by the elderly eases the strain on families of limited means.

The older person in the US and UK may be pictured as someone to be taken care of rather than someone who is self-sufficient or who cares for others. This may be far from the truth. Old parents may continue to give more to their children than they receive, according to a West German survey.

There is great loss of self-esteem among the elderly in countries where gross dependency is the prevalent image. There is often a corresponding lack of respect for the elderly by the younger generations, a serious problem in the UK and the US. Rapid improvement in educational levels has contributed to a great cultural gap between older and younger persons, say several countries' experts.

The experts note that the trend towards women in paid employment has intensified the concept that all worthwhile adults must engage in paid work. At the same time, the trend removes caretakers from the home, and they must be replaced or the sick person institutionalized.

The UK experts say that 30 years of the welfare state has lulled people into thinking that all of their needs and those of their elderly relatives will be met. Individuals may not set aside money for the later years. The concept that families should care for their elderly relatives is fading. With increased longevity, say the UK experts, the generation caring for the oldest will itself be from 60 to 70 years of age, and may be too weak, tired, or disinclined to care for their relatives aged 85 or 90. Social systems in the UK have developed largely to care for older people without families, not to support the families struggling to care for their own relatives.

Swedish experts assert that the cost of an improved standard of living has been an impoverished and weakened family unit. Support for the elderly from the general community becomes necessary.

Programs and policies today

Almost all the more developed countries have some kinds of family-support programs vis-a-vis the elderly. The experts believe these programs do not provide adequate direct or indirect financial aid or services.

West German experts report that home helps, social centers, health insurance for home nursing, day clinics, and a few guest beds in nursing homes are available. But the experts believe much more needs to be done.

Israel, with unusual problems due to immigration, has only limited home help and home health-care. The experts say, however, that financial assistance is offered to each needy immigrant.

Kenyan experts say there are virtually no programs. A few community centers have developed on a private basis with the understanding that those who live in the area will help either financially or via services. They hope that rural improvement programs will help keep young people in rural areas, and so limit the isolation of the elderly.

The Philippines offers both government and privately run family counseling centers, as well as vocational training for the elderly. Their self-employment assistance program offers no-interest, no-collateral loans for the elderly who want to begin income-generating projects, such as small farms to raise chickens, vending operations, or craft enterprises.

The UK experts report a program of allowances to families who spend 35 hours a week caring for their elderly relatives. This is basically a token payment, rather than a salary equivalent. Sweden, supporting such allowances in principle, has not yet been able to institute such a program.

The US has no real policies or programs in this area. The experts are pessimistic that any will develop soon. Help for families caring for elderly relatives tends in the US to come from voluntary associations and from fragmented public and private income-maintenance programs. Family life is changing so rapidly in the United States that a recent White House Conference on the Family, in December 1979, was unable to agree on a definition of "the family".

Japanese experts cite government efforts to bolster the spirit of independence among the old. Various changes have been made in Japanese civil laws to equalize the inheritance rights of children and allow women to vote. The experts say that "the elderly still lack the spirit of individual independence."

The year 2000

In urbanized countries, the family will adapt to conditions of longer lives along new and, from the standpoint of parent and older-child relationships, possibly more supportive lines by the year 2000. Less developed countries fear dissolution of the family and abandonment of the elderly. Decline in family support of the elderly is expected in India. Kenyan commentators expect that total collapse of the extended family system will isolate many of the rural elders. Foreign influence is a destructive force, say Filipino experts, who fear erosion of indigenous values. They foresee that ideological change and materialism will undermine care of the elderly.

Family breakdown at all levels will continue in the UK. Divorce, re-marriage, and informal cohabitation will lessen the commitment to take care of older relatives just when families extend into four and five generations.

Financial issues are cited by the US experts as ominous. Inflation will make many older people financially dependent. Furthermore, many childless couples will have no one to help them in their old age. Housing costs will make it difficult for those who do have children to live with them in multi-generational units.

The US experts see more and more people over age 80. Two out of three will be women, and the vast majority will be widowed. Many of their children will be about 55–60 years of age.

Italian and Israeli experts note optimistically that the older generation will be better educated; this will help family relationships by narrowing inter-generational gaps. Italian respondents urge an approach to the elderly that falls between a "gerontocracy" and marginalism. They envision a "solidarity" approach which would create a society where everybody, regardless of age, will have a role and a function. They would encourage a "neo-matriarchal society", with the grandmother rearing the children and the younger parents banding together to work in cooperatives and free to move in search of work. In any case they see the elderly, by the year 2000, as having more financial resources than do the elderly today.

Recommendations

New roles for the elderly are needed, say many of the international experts. These should be developed through assessment of social roles, continued employment, volunteer work, child care, and other services needed by a community or a family. The young as well as the elderly should be educated to assume these new roles. The media can be helpful, say many experts, in promoting new images of old age.

Experts from Israel, the UK, and Sweden stress that many of the problems of the elderly would be solved if every older person would be financially independent. A minimum income and continued right to work are the means suggested to promote a dignified position for the older member in a family.

Israeli experts articulate a major theme in the concept of shared care of the elderly. Experts from many countries feel that this is an important idea. Israelis are studying various forms of assistance to the elderly and their families, to determine which are the most helpful. Among the types of assistance they are investigating are:

- tax relief for families with elderly relatives
- vouchers for necessities of the elderly
- giving the people who support the elderly added vacation time from work, similar to the leave granted parents of small children.

Experts from various countries, notably the UK, urge assistance to families caring for the frail elderly. They suggest respite programs, emergency assistance, and holiday relief programs.

Kenyan experts would urge communities to take care of the elderly – even those not from their own area. Nigerian experts believe stabilization of family life will eventually help the elderly.

Filipino experts advocate campaigns to support traditional values, such as respect for the elderly and their wisdom and close family ties. They would also teach young people how to save for their own later years.

Egypt would advise more funds to their program for supporting the setting-up of income-generating enterprises for the elderly.

Measures on the US list include a change in image for the elderly: the creation of new family-like groups (group living) for those who are isolated; expanded employment opportunities; new forms of public and private income maintenance insurance and health insurance financed outside the systems now in place; and research on aging, particularly on the serious problem of senile dementia.

Swedish recommendations look to systems that link assessment of the individual's and family's socio-economic and other needs to a wide spectrum of deliverable services in communities and institutions. A strong emphasis should be placed on encouraging the elderly to remain active. Activity would increase an overall sense of well-being, the experts say.

Chapter 7

THE INDIVIDUAL AND THE COMMUNITY

Order of priority given to "Community":

1	KENYA		
2			
3	FRANCE	NIGERIA	
4	EGYPT		
5	BRAZIL	ISRAEL	ITALY
6	AUSTRALIA	UK	
7	JAPAN	SWEDEN	
8	PHILIPPINES	USA	
9	W. GERMANY	INDIA	POLAND

The problems today

In many countries, old people are considered burdensome, obsolete, and virtually useless. This negative image, common in the majority of countries surveyed, produces apathy on the part of the elderly and those around them toward roles and supports for elders by the community. In some countries, communities themselves have lost a sense of identity and neighborliness, owing to industrialization and urbanization. The elderly tend to be misunderstood and unsupported in urban communities that hardly have a life of their own.

The elderly deprecate themselves, lack confidence, and have narrow interests, say the West German experts. The French experts say that aging is misconceived as unalloyed decline, even though there is lifelong growth in creative, conceptual, and other faculties. In Sweden, the elderly are patronized, almost infantilized: although lacking a community role and encouraged to be inactive, they are supplied in the community with health, social, and other services.

A tendency to accord the elderly no participatory role in community, government, or voluntary organizations is seen in the UK. Fear of gerontocracy is cited. Policies concerning housing and environmental conditions, say the UK experts, impede traditional kinds of community support; they isolate the generations and disperse formerly tight-knit communities.

Nigerian experts report that the elderly retain respected roles in communities. The Kenyans find the elderly neglected, socially isolated, and in conflict with the young. General economic distress in Kenya has undermined a collective spirit in communities; every family is out for itself, and the elderly have nothing to do.

A strong community spirit is evident in rural India, where the elderly retain traditional roles. In urban India, however, their roles are unclear and they get far less support than in the hinterland.

Inter-generational conflict and orientation to youth are coupled with social isolation of the elderly in several nations: the Philippines, Kenya, Australia, Italy, and the US are among them. In Israel, the "founding father" generation of elders appears far more active than the elders who came later. But both waves encounter young activists who are ousting the elderly from leadership. The survivors of World War II, many of whom have no children or other relatives in Israel, are especially isolated and lonely in a youth-oriented society.

Many US communities are slow to consider supports for the elderly, largely in the mistaken belief that they are well off. At the same time, the elderly are regarded as deviants, being non-workers and sick. Crime against the elderly is noted along with their isolation, reflecting community indifference. However, there are wealthy elders who can retreat to safe but isolated "golden ghettoes".

The loss of work role in Japan leaves the male urban elder virtually without community status or function. So much effort has been invested in life as an employee that the retired worker has no developed interest in the community. In Poland, few community organizations support the elderly, and they face an urban environment filled with architectural and social barriers.

According to the Australian experts, the elderly have no clear roles in their communities, which are indifferent to them. Support for local services varies among jurisdictions and categories of aid. Government subsidies to communities are not indexed to inflation, so that the supply of domiciliary services declines as the population grows.

The isolation of the elderly is a result of both community and self attitudes. Keeping to themselves makes the elderly ignorant of the community, the Australian experts say. Egyptian commentators point out that incentives are lacking for elderly participation in community life. Apartment living, new to many of the Japanese elderly, tends to separate retirees from their families, while providing no structure for community and other social involvement.

Policies and programs today

Many of the more developed countries report a varied list of official and volunteer community services. Often they are only token, poorly financed, and poorly coordinated. To the extent the elderly participate in delivering these services, they acquire community roles as givers rather than receivers. Senior centers furnish both roles and services for the elderly in some countries. Some experts cite discount prices for transportation and cultural or entertainment activities in their lists of community services.

In the UK, service to the community has become part of schooling and programs for teenagers. Local authorities promote "good neighbor schemes", and street wardens provide informal care and supervision of the elderly. Pensioner groups for cooperative aid have been set up by community workers, and Age Concern volunteers offer visiting, counseling, and other services.

The US elderly may find opportunities to remain socially active through foster grandparent, retired executive, and other volunteer programs.

The West German list of services available in communities includes meals, home helps, body care, shopping, advice, visiting, escort and wheelchair, mobile libraries, house cleaning, excursions, community day care, recreation, and rehabilitation. By contrast, India reports no formal programs specifically for the elderly.

Education for elders or involving the elderly with children occurs in several lands. In the US, community colleges promote lifelong education, and the elders are organized to assist in local schools. Some UK schools encourage the elderly to contribute to courses on local history.

Israel fosters inter-generational encounters through youth movements and schools. Considerable aid is organized by local Associations for the Aged, which plan and conduct social action programs. The associations include lay and professional persons, representatives of agencies serving the elderly, public figures, and the elderly. There also are associations that support local leaders in lobbying at the national level for the elderly.

According to the Italian experts, today's elders are separated from youth because of poor education in the past. For future Italian elderly people, this barrier will not exist.

The importance of television for the elderly is cited in more developed and less developed countries. Egyptian television has a program that brings information and advice to the elderly, and seeks to improve inter-generational understanding and grass-roots awareness of problems of the elderly.

Australia has Councils on the Aged, which produce literature and seminars on age prejudice and promote participation in community activities. However, the aged who participate tend to be those individuals who were doers all their lives. Japan has Corporations for the Aged, which organize small commercial activities by the elderly and assist in referring the elderly to jobs for which they have the skills. Poland is trying to add to day-care centers, senior clubs, and old-age homes.

The year 2000

Problems concerning roles and supports for the elderly in their communities are unlikely to be resolved by the year 2000, according to many experts. The problems may even worsen.

Government is unlikely to increase support substantially in Australia, and communities there will continue to view the elderly as drains on their resources. The US elders may become scapegoats for economic frustrations in American society, but also may develop political awareness and power to improve their situation. The same may occur in Italy.

Increased indifference to the elderly in the Philippines, India, and Nigeria will accompany modernization. More elderly persons will be living alone in Israel, increasing expectations and pressures on community services. Sweden may lack practitioners versed in geriatrics and gerontology.

Further decline of neighborly support is seen in the UK, where a balanced social fabric is not expected to arise without broad initiatives in the fields of housing, employment, and social services. Loosening of ties between the elderly and communities is foreseen in Egypt, as cities become more over-crowded and their people, more engrossed in their own problems, less able to assist others. The generation gap in Egypt, as in other countries, is expected to widen.

In West Germany, conflict between active and inactive elders is conceivable: the go-go's, slow-go's, and no-go's have divergent interests. Political activity by pensioner associations will grow in Sweden as competition for community resources increases. In the Philippines, the elderly may be excluded from community decision-making roles; in urban India, they will be shunted aside; the Italian elderly may find ways to get the services they will demand; and people generally will acquire a new understanding of aging.

Recommendations

The experts would like policies to strengthen the community roles of the elderly through paid employment, education of the young and old in problems of aging, changes in community and elderly attitudes, promotion of inter-generational encounters, and development of services, particularly volunteer services, in which the elderly may participate.

In terms of supports by the community, the experts suggest that communities themselves be strengthened, that the elderly become aware of their political weight, that neighborliness be promoted with incentives, and that work be re-allocated across the lifespan.

Government pump-priming of community services is a Japanese recommendation. The Brazilians and Japanese call for the elderly to be represented on the institutions that serve them. The Australians, Japanese, and Egyptians, among others, recommend more preparation for non-work activities and more programs to stimulate the elderly. However, a relatively new country or community may develop a leadership cohort ("founding fathers") at a particular time in its history. The positions held by such a cohort, now elderly, should not necessarily be reserved for elderly persons, the Israeli experts point out. To attempt to do so may produce only palliative or cosmetic results, especially when young activists challenge a fading gerontocracy. Some role changes may even be desirable.

Calls for integrating the elderly into their communities are sounded by experts in various countries, notably Brazil, Israel, and Nigeria. The US experts would eliminate age as a criterion in government assistance programs; ability to pay should replace it. Work and leisure time should be re-distributed over the lifespan under a plan worked up by a federal body. The US also should develop a domestic Peace Corps of old and young volunteers, create job opportunities for the elderly, and encourage communities to support group medical practices for the aged.

Voluntary agencies in India should develop community centers, to provide education on aging as well as recreation and health services. Improved financial support would help the elderly to maintain independence and freedom of choice, the UK experts add.

The Italians suggest the study of primitive societies to see how roles and tasks might be adjusted according to age. The Poles would study the environment to identify and correct barriers to participation by the elderly in community life, and conditions favoring remaining in their own homes rather than being institutionalized.

The most frequent recommendation concerns attitudinal change, specifically elimination of age prejudice. The Swedes want reform of professional as well as lay attitudes. The Filipinos would encourage "value revival", bolstered by the formation of Councils of Elders as community and institutional advisors. The Nigerian experts also would strengthen traditional concepts and social organization.

Getting children to realize that elders are important is a Japanese objective, along with creation of jobs for the elderly in education, social welfare, and health care in the community.

Chapter 8

LEISURE ACTIVITIES AND THE USE OF TIME

Order of priority given to "Activities and the use of time":

1				
2	FRANCE			
3	SWEDEN			
4	W GERMANY	JAPAN		
5				
6	POLAND	UK		
7	AUSTRALIA	ITALY	NIGERIA	
8	BRAZIL	INDIA	ISRAEL	KENYA
9	EGYPT	PHILIPPINES	USA	

The main problems today

"Retirement is the real cause of aging."

The words of A. M. Guillemard are quoted by the French experts in stating the problems as perceived in their country. It is noteworthy that the French experts identify "activities and the use of time" as the second most important issue on a list ranging from health and provision of services to housing and income (see figure above).

Whether "retirement" is taken to mean removal from the work-force or from organized leisure, the view that idleness means social death is shared by many of the experts in the surveyed countries. Yet, no strong tradition exists for the use of free time creatively in many of the same countries, including Israel, West Germany, and the US. The American experts observe that apathy of the elderly, and their discouragement by society in developing leisure-time pursuits, are outgrowths of widespread prejudice against "selfish" use of time, as opposed to time used constructively for society.

A reinforcing sequence of attitudes and actions leading to social death are described by the Australian experts. Boredom and resignation are apparent in many elderly persons unused to free-time pursuits. These attitudes become barriers to effective use of free time. Feeling unwanted, the elderly retreat from social activities.

According to the Egyptians, older people believe that old age is a time of inability, and nobody contradicts them. The Polish elderly turn to television, spending little time in active recreation, social life, and political activities. The West Germans say that watching TV bars the development of social and creative activities among the elders.

Among less developed nations, like India, Kenya, and Nigeria, a need for formal assistance to the elderly in organizing leisure time is becoming recognized, but no consensus has formed on how to meet it.

The possibility that problems experienced by today's elderly may not be the same for future birth cohorts in old age is raised by experts from several countries. Improved educational levels and new life-styles may make a difference in leisure time usage for future elders. The Polish experts note that old age will be influenced by how the individual organized his time earlier in life, and the West German experts say that a person's old-age patterns are established in youth. The West Germans also note that today's middle-aged lack time, opportunity, and motivation to develop non-work activities, although the young have the incentives. The UK experts point out that today's elders have not been trained for leisure.

As the American experts suggest, cultivation of non-work activities is not taken seriously throughout the life-cycle.

Some respondents took the issue of "activities and use of time" to mean work as well as non-work activities. The Japanese cite needs for jobs and needs for opportunities, through adult education, to develop new skills and careers. The Kenyan and Egyptian experts include employment as an "activities" need, and they note inadequate facilities for recreation, continuing education, and opportunities for service in advisory and counseling roles.

Lack of money is a barrier to pursuing non-work or leisure interests, according to the Israelis. The history of today's elderly, as well as their income status, helps to explain their weak leisure interests. The opportunity to develop them in earlier life was lacking for many elderly Israelis, because they immigrated to a country where the work week is six days and two jobs are often needed for survival.

In sum, the major problems are rooted in "ageism", or negative attitudes toward the elderly and old age, poor recognition of the retiree's need for non-work interests, and lack of facilities and programs for developing such interests among elders and the young.

Policies and programs

All the sampled countries except India report some organized leisure activities for the elderly. According to the Indian experts, no formal policies and programs exist for the constructive use of leisure time, though there are informal groups in urban and rural areas for this purpose.

In the main, programs in the other countries appear to be token, scarce, or underdeveloped when measured against needs and demands. In some countries, programs sponsored by voluntary groups (religious, philanthropic, and senior citizen bodies, organized by area or by former work relationship) seem to be more elaborate than those developed governmentally, at least those developed by the national government.

This appears to be the case in the United Kingdom, where the experts find national government policies to be minimal, while voluntary organizations and local authorities support a variety of clubs, day centers, and educational activities.

Many retirees in the UK work as volunteers in service to other elderly persons. One scheme, Link Opportunity, organizes retirees to exchange services for credits and thus conserve their cash incomes. Similar plans have appeared, the sponsors say, in Ireland, Australia, New Zealand, Canada, the United States, and Belgium. A local group does the administration, and makes clear to trade unions that the work performed by retirees does not reduce paid work opportunities for the union members.

Television programs are produced specially for the elderly in the UK and other countries, with mixed implications for promoting socialization. Some experts believe that television in general reinforces passivity and seclusion. For example, some elderly viewers who might leave their houses to attend sports events may remain at home and watch the events on TV. Some elderly persons, fearing crime in the streets, depend heavily on TV for entertainment. The experts also note that the medium offers useful information and instruction.

Programs of adult education figure heavily in meeting leisure needs of the elderly in a number of countries. In France and Poland, "Universities of the Third Age" have been organized for the elderly. In Japan, colleges for the aged exist in some communities. The United States has educational programs for the elderly based in universities and community colleges.

In several countries, elders receive reduced-rate tickets to cultural, spectator sports, and recreational events. Reduced-rate transportation within a locality, or for national and international tourism, may be found in a number of countries. Large groups of wealthier retirees in the United States provide their own travel services.

Senior citizen centers and community centers are sites for leisure activities and headquarters for mutual assistance in various countries. The Polish experts report that centers for the well elderly have grown fourfold in the last five years; they provide educational and cultural benefits along with meals and medical care.

The American observers make note of the private sector production of leisure-time goods and services; although mainly for younger people, these goods and services occasionally are prepared specifically for older people.

As for the use of leisure time by the elderly for service to society in general, the Italian experts note attempts to involve elders in private social welfare organizations, religious and political groups, child care activities, and consulting to former employers. The US government helps retired executives to organize as consultants to novice businessmen, and it helps to support foster grandparent and other volunteer service to society.

Japan has Corporations for the Aged, which are small businesses operated by the elderly and producing handicrafts or offering services. According to Swedish experts, public authorities in their country make no effort to keep the elderly in their accustomed occupations when they reach retirement age, but promote a variety of recreational activities. The Polish observers describe their countrymen as mistrustful of institutions, and therefore unlikely to accept formal offerings of free-time activities.

In the Philippines, Brazil, Egypt, and India, no planned activities or only a token number are reported for the elderly population. The Nigerian experts say that problems in the use of leisure time have not emerged on any large scale, and no programs or policies exist specifically for the aged.

Only the American experts comment on programs in middle age and earlier to orient people toward leisure or non-work activities. They find only a smattering of work-sabbatical programs in corporations. Some corporations offer educational benefits to their pensioners.

The year 2000

Problems noted in the preparation for, and use of, leisure time will persist, if not deepen, in the next 20 years, according to many of the experts.

If unemployment and earlier retirement trends intensify, as some expect, the need to develop non-work interests and to organize and support leisure activities will grow apace. How will idleness and its

117

accompaniments of boredom, anxiety, and frustration be met? Occupational re-training? Voluntary service? Recreational opportunities? The answers are mixed and hedged.

Some experts see the elderly populations as demanding more of public and private resources, thereby generating further inter-generational conflict (Japan, US). Some foresee development of a leisure time industry catering to the elders as they acquire pensions along with free time (Israel, US). Some see expanding demand for old workers in part-time work (Poland).

The Swedish experts distinguish between the well elders, who are generally younger, and the frail elders, generally very old. New kinds of occupations probably will be devised for the well elders who are unable to keep up with technological changes. For the very old, the problem will be to find ways of keeping them active. Many of them will be living alone and will lack education and experience to use their abundant free time.

Among the less developed countries, such as Egypt, extension of both life expectancy and unemployment is foreseen. The elders will recognize a need to develop useful interests. In Brazil's struggling economy, the elders will be adrift – with neither employment nor support for leisure activities. In India, urban elders will be hard put to find useful activities for their spare time. Kenya sees a future with more loneliness among the elders and social distress among the young. Needs will intensify in the Philippines for educational, sports, and recreational activities for the elders.

The Italian experts believe that younger elders will be idle and alienated, ripe for exploitation by vendors of squalid and uninspiring "entertainment". In the UK, leisure facilities will be needed for the elderly and the unemployed, while in Australia, where earlier retirement is expected, leisure programs will be swamped by the demand and may be, in effect, rationed so that everyone may have some access to them.

The Japanese experts believe that a "culture of the aged" will develop as this population grows. There will be more energetic retirees. The issue will be to turn their leisure into an asset for the country.

Recommendations

Proposals fall into several main categories:

1. Training of older persons for public-sector jobs in social assistance to persons of all ages.

2. Training for private-sector jobs, including part-time work and positions specially adapted to capacities of the elderly person.

3. Development of services and facilities to assist the elderly in personal development and satisfaction.

4. Life-cycle programs to orient people to non-work activities and satisfactions.

The experts' recommendations often do not specify the agencies or sectors responsible for devising and implementing the proposals. But it appears that no one places responsibility solely on government, business, or other agency. A variety of agencies must act, as well as the elders themselves.

The Indian accent is on developing community programs. The Brazilians suggest creating leisure activity organizations, such as cooperatives and cottage industries. The West Germans urge participation in recreational activities beginning in youth. The Australians call for consultant roles for the elders, and the formation of job and skill inventories to help place the elderly.

The British and Italians want lifelong programs of education and training, and the Americans want jobs to be structured to allow for more and more non-work activities as retirement approaches. The British prescription for lifelong education features informality, self-direction, and the use of television.

Roles for employers are often suggested, mainly for pre-retirement training in which employees learn about services, benefits, health and social needs, and lifestyles of later life. The Israeli experts propose that employers design pre-retirement programs in collaboration with worker representatives and outside experts, that trade unions encourage members to participate, and that aged associations provide speakers to discuss experiences in adjusting to retirement.

The Poles propose that government require business and other enterprises to reserve certain jobs – typically allowing for less than full time or effort – for the elderly. Leisure time counseling also should be available. The Americans believe job counseling should be offered at senior centers, as well as through personnel departments of businesses.

The Egyptians concentrate on education and volunteer work. They propose that the government promote the use of elderly volunteers in local social services. Schools should use retired teachers to make up for the emigration of young teachers to other countries. Universities should open courses to the elderly so they may learn skills and new vocations.

In a broad set of recommendations, the Japanese call for training of the elderly for jobs in social welfare, education, and public facilities, such as libraries and museums; enlisting the elderly as trainers of new workers at their old work-places; and encouraging old people's clubs to adopt recreational and educational objectives.

Perhaps the most systematic approach is suggested by the Swedish experts. They are alone in calling for scientific intervention studies to test means of continuing older persons at work and utilizing them in volunteer and other activities, on a full-time or part-time basis. The urban environment must be modified to enable the elderly to live independently, especially by facilitating their access to libraries, theaters, public services, and other destinations. A particular plea is made for special programs to help the elderly "catch up" with the educational level of younger generations. For example, while one-third of persons aged 20–40 have a college education, only 3–4% of those aged 70 or more have one.

In general, the experts seek solutions: to lack of training for leisure, not only among the elders but also among their juniors; to the deadening effect of, and growing absorption in, television; and to the apathy of elderly persons toward forms of active leisure.

Chapter 9

EMPLOYMENT

Order of priority given to "Employment":

1	FRANCE	JAPAN			
2	BRAZIL	INDIA			
3	PHILIPPINES	USA			
4					
5	SWEDEN				
6	W. GERMANY	ISRAEL	KENYA	NIGERIA	
7					
8	AUSTRALIA	EGYPT	ITALY	POLAND	UK
9					

The main problems today

The characteristic unemployment problems of older workers – including policies to move them out of the work-force even when they are able and willing to continue – derive basically from a shortage of jobs for persons of all ages, in the view of most experts in the Sandoz Institute survey. This generic shortage occurs in both the less and more developed lands. It reflects rates of population growth as well as industrialization.

The experts see age prejudice, and unwillingness to adapt hours and work circumstances to the needs and capacities of older workers, as reasons why older workers tend to be dismissed from the available job pool or not hired. In many countries, unemployment even before age 50 becomes chronic and, in effect, retirement. When retirees are covered poorly or not at all by social insurance or pension programs, they suffer impoverishment and may sink into destitution.

Also observed with concern are social insurance policies that entirely or substantially discourage earnings after retirement. For example, in the Unites States and Australia, cash benefits are reduced when earnings exceed a limit. The justification for such actions is that retirement programs are intended to make jobs available to younger workers who have growing families.

Although this policy appears to accommodate the young, it carries a burden that grows with improvements in life expectancy. Most social insurance and pension programs were established at a time when average life expectancy was less than it is today. The additional years of life remaining after conventional retirement age have funding implications. More taxes or contributions must be paid during the working years of the future retiree, or by today's working population, for today's retirees. Especially in a period of inflation, the strain on workers to pay for retirement grows. The responding experts generally see this strain as a source of inter-generational hostility. They see no easing – indeed, they typically see a worsening – by the year 2000.

Pressure for earlier retirement stems from the "baby boom" that followed World War II, the Italian gerontologists note. They and other commentators in western industrialized countries indicate that employment policies favored by trade unions produce high wages at the expense of novices and pensioners. Employers in several countries act as though the older worker is less efficient than the younger worker; actually, ability to perform in many occupations is unaffected by age until perhaps very late life.

Inflation was perceived as both a reason why elderly workers need employment and why younger workers want them out of the work-force.

Because work is a central psychosocial pivot of life, retirement and employment policies have profound extra-economic implications. Whether intended or not, such policies contribute to the way in which the older person sees himself or herself, and the way in which society looks at the older person. Typically, the elderly are devalued in what French commentators called their "pensioned idleness". These prejudices may be self-fulfilling. The contemporary view of the elderly as necessarily sick, or having unreliable health and ability, reflects age prejudice and promotes pauperization through exclusion from gainful employment. Pauperization contributes to depression or exacerbates illness. There rarely are opportunities for working oneself out of chronic poverty in later life. Expectation of dependency invites the behavior. In some countries, it may even be easier to play the sick role than to strive for independence.

To meet inflation, some elderly workers seek part-time employment. In some countries, jobs with flexible hours are available but are scarce. Employers are seen as rarely willing to adapt jobs to the abilities and needs of the elderly.

A contrast between more developed and less developed countries exists in the perception of older-worker employment problems. For example, here is a summary of an Australian view:

Older unemployed workers have trouble finding jobs. While the government insists on means-testing of pensions as a measure to control spending, means-testing creates a disincentive to part-time work, even though a job helps pensioners maintain mental and physical well-being. Not enough jobs with flexible hours are available in the private sector. Pressure exists for earlier retirement, but alternatives to full retirement are lacking.

And the view from Poland:

Because of unemployment, the retirement age is inflexible. Retirees face difficult economic, psychological, and social problems: rapid pauperization, being ignored by former colleagues and neighbors, and rapid loss of social position. Jobs that are available are physically taxing, beyond the strength of retirees. Many needs persist in retirement but resources are lacking, especially among laborers and clerks, for meeting them.

And from India:

Unemployment is a major national problem. Most workers only have part-time work. Rural employment is seasonal. The elderly rarely have job opportunities.

Policies and programs today

Several countries report programs for vocational re-training of the older worker, but these appear to be on a small scale (e.g. Japan, UK, West Germany) or frankly token (Brazil). Job placement programs are in operation in Israel, but are under-used. In other countries, employees may request extension of the retirement age (e.g. the Philippines). Public sector jobs adapted to the older worker are provided in Sweden. In West Germany, the concept of phased retirement is being introduced. Egypt has a limited program for teaching the elderly income-generating crafts in day-care centers.

Perhaps the greatest variety of programs is reported for the United States, though the experts say the programs generally do not meet the problems adequately. For example, re-training programs are treated as charity rather than as human investment. A law against age discrimination is just beginning to be tested.

The year 2000

By and large, the experts see employment prospects worsening for the older worker in the coming two decades. Scant relaxation of mandatory retirement is foreseen. More early retirement is considered likely. While older workers step aside for younger workers in job-shrinking economies, the conventional-age working population is expected to bridle at the costs of maintaining the elderly population. Sweden sees a chance that competition for jobs might lead to job-sharing, with the elders included. West Germany sees more unemployed elderly as a consequence of industrial standardization. However, Italy sees improvement in employment of the elderly as a consequence of declining birth rates.

Brazil sees itself falling behind other national economies; it has only scarce programs to re-train workers for new technologies. Egypt, Nigeria, and India see population growth outstripping job growth, with elderly joblessness aggravated. In the United States, skilled workers born in the Great Depression of the 1930s, a low birth-rate cohort, will be in short supply and probably will have little difficulty in staying at work if they wish.

Recommendations

Expansion of national economies to achieve full employment appears to be implied, where not made explicit, by the experts as necessary to solving problems of employment and income maintenance among the elderly. (Japan puts at 5% the annual growth needed in the economy to ease elderly unemployment.)

A shortage of jobs is recognized as exacerbating young-old hostilities. The possibility of creating jobs outside the private sector is raised by experts from several countries. Accommodating the elderly to jobs (by re-training, second careers) and the reverse (by re-designing jobs and work-places) are proposed.

In the absence of full employment, a cluster of proposals aim at sharing work throughout the lifespan by sabbaticals, part-time jobs, and shorter hours. (Such an approach would mean flattening the life-income curve.) To add to employment possibilities for the elderly without threatening jobs for others (at least directly), there are proposals for promoting craft, artisan, and small business opportunities. There is some concern that automation will reduce the availability of jobs, and one country (Brazil) explicitly calls for the creation of labor-intensive occupations to counterbalance industrial automation.

Yet another set of proposals aims at prohibiting mandatory retirement and lower retirement ages than those now in effect, or to promote later retirement, both for the sake of easing the impact of inflation on the elderly and their pension funds and for continuing the social and psychological benefits of employment. Here is a roll call of proposals:

1. Spreading work and leisure through the adult population (West Germany, UK, Japan, US).

2. Phased retirement, abandoning mandatory retirement by practice or statute, and/or extension of retirement age beyond 65 (UK, Japan, Philippines, Poland).

(a) Legislation to prohibit lowering the retirement age (Philippines).

(b) Meaningful work throughout the adult years as a matter of right, and disregard of age as a basic qualification for a pension (Sweden).

3. Designing jobs and work-places to meet needs of the elderly, including flexible hours and part-time arrangements (Poland, West Germany, Egypt).

4. Providing lifetime access to training for private and public sector work, including unpaid community work and paid work as advisors (Brazil, Israel, West Germany, Kenya).

5. Creating volunteer occupations (US, specifically a National Corps of Youth and Aging) and orienting people in youth for such work in retirement (Japan).

6. Establishing inventories of jobs and skills to help the elderly find work (Egypt).

7. Eliminating barriers to earnings by pensioners (US, Australia).

8. Assisting establishment of small business and artisan enterprises (cottage industries) by and for the elderly (Australia, Brazil, India).

9. Encouraging barter of goods and services among the elderly (Australia).

10. Encouraging corporations to participate in community improvement, and use of the elderly in such work (Japan).

11. Awarding pensions on basis of need, not age (Italy), or studying an income-test approach (US).

Noteworthy are: the Australian comment that people should be prepared for aging, not retirement; the Japanese suggestion that, beginning in youth, people should be prepared for retirement; the UK view that work-sharing, which also means leisure-sharing, would have a beneficial effect in blurring the retirement/employment dichotomy; the Egyptian view that promotion of the economy and of family planning are of significance to the elderly, and that the elderly worker, before retirement, should receive special training in new skills; and the Israeli concept that career change be an accepted part of a comprehensive long-term employment policy.

Chapter 10

PREPARATION FOR RETIREMENT

The main problems today

Retirement must be prepared for during the entire working career, according to most experts in the Sandoz Institute survey. Indeed, many go beyond by saying that an understanding of physical, mental, and social aging should be incorporated into the public education of children and youth and reinforced during the working years.

Preparation, therefore, is not fundamentally as much for retirement as it is for aging. It is the individual as a whole being, rather than the individual as a worker, who must prepare, and be assisted in preparing, for coping with major experiences of life.

Although this concept may appear remote from what is ordinarily presumed to be retirement preparation, its adoption by policy-makers and program planners in public and private sectors is strongly advocated. Whatever is done by employers at the work-place to orient workers to retirement must be supplemented and even prepared for by schools, higher education, the mass media, church and other mutual support groups, and other activities.

Against this concept, the practices and attitudes that prevent a blending of retirement leisure activity into the working lifetime are seen by the experts as problems. Similarly, some experts view social emphasis on immediate consumption as a serious threat to apportioning work income across the lifespan, including a larger investment into pensions and other mechanisms for supporting retirement. This latter concern, dealt with in Chapter 11 on income maintenance in retirement, must be mentioned here at least superficially in terms of retirement preparation.

In many experts' comments is an implied observation that the work role has been so heavily stressed that when it is abandoned — willingly or not — the individual is devalued. The person who was a good "consumer" finds, in retirement at reduced income, that he or she no longer is "good" or desired. The loss of good consumer status also afflicts individuals at any age who become so severely ill that they cannot earn an adequate income. Indeed, prejudice against the elderly may become so ingrained in the younger individual that,

127

when he or she becomes older, the prejudice is self-prejudice. To avoid identification with being older and retired, many workers avoid retirement preparation, some experts observe. This, too, is a fundamental problem in many nations.

The French experts are emphatic that retirement preparation and preparation for aging are intertwined. Aging preparation is the more encompassing objective. From the social planning viewpoint, it should take precedence; it concerns everyone, not just those in paid work or about to leave it. Preparing for aging, say the French respondents, means extending the skills one should have in managing life throughout its course, as best one can, particularly husbanding resources and optimizing possibilities of making satisfying adaptations to changing needs. The circumstances that engage such skills include career, parenthood, marriage, sickness, disability, widowhood, one's own approaching death, and one's participation in community, religious, leisure, and volunteer activities.

Even in countries with the most sophisticated pre-retirement perspectives, many future pensioners are ignorant about benefits, services, and needs. For example, according to Swedish respondents, only one-third of future pensioners believe they are adequately informed about their pensions. Many acknowledge ignorance of housing and rental allowances. More important in the eyes of Swedish experts is ignorance of processes of aging; specifically, what to expect in old age when one is healthy or sick, how to compensate for losses and maximize residual abilities, and when to seek assistance and preventive measures.

The US experts note that most of those in need of information on how to prepare for retirement, and what benefits and services to expect, are least likely to get adequate education or training. This results from the fact that preparation is mistakenly assigned only to the period just before retirement. Moreover, the training or educational efforts are relatively superficial.

In Brazil, as in other countries, many people do not know what to do with their leisure time, and programs for utilizing leisure time may be absent or lack appeal.

In many countries, it appears that most individuals – except for participation in pension and social insurance schemes – make no systematic retirement preparations and fail to demand programs that will inform them. Orientation programs may be entirely lacking, available only to a narrow segment of the population, or existing in fragments.

What possible reasons are there for the absence of demand for retirement information? One is a negative view of retirement. The

United Kingdom commentators find that men resent retirement because of the loss of masculine work role, the implied feminization that they see awaiting them in post-retirement domestication, and — overall — a bleak perception of retirement life and the loss of work-based friendships.

The abruptness of retirement — "retirement shock", to use a phrase supplied by Egyptian observers — is widespread among individuals and families in some countries. The phenomenon evinces the need for retirement preparation, the experts say. In Japan, this recognition is growing but it is unclear which institution should take the lead in meeting the need. In a number of countries, responsibility for systematizing pre-retirement preparation has yet to be accepted or assigned in public and private sectors.

Policies and programs today

Some measures are being taken to provide retirement preparation, to at least some groups, in most countries. No country appears to have a national policy on retirement preparation as a whole, but there are scattered systems. For example, federal workers in the United States are offered pre-retirement orientation in a one-day program offered on government time. But the program can only be considered introductory.

Perhaps the most systematic national attempt at retirement preparation appears in Israel. In 1975, the ministry of labor established the National Authority on Retirees and on Preparation for Retirement, as a result of various government and trade union studies. Preparatory programs are of recent vintage. They are conducted on company time and expense, covering — in a few meetings — retirement benefits, health problems, legal matters, and leisure time use. Few elderly persons make plans for retirement, the Israeli experts note, but a growing number see a need. A survey showed that 7% of companies had a pre-retirement program and 67% exhibited interest in having one. The primary concern of pre-retirees is income maintenance.

In the US and Sweden, information useful in preparing for retirement may be forthcoming in fragments, during youth employment counseling, discussion of health maintenance and life-insurance programs, and participation in recreational programs. In union negotiations for retirement benefits, the rank-and-file membership may become educated on needs and issues. The US experts say that a few programs develop lifecycle informational materials for use with young people.

Information on what to expect in retirement comes to Swedes in fragmented fashion, through social welfare, social insurance, housing, labor, and other national organizations; through municipalities and county councils; through education and pension associations; through county colleges; and through employers and unions. Proposals for coordinating the delivery of retirement information have been made in Sweden.

Similar patterns of fragmented delivery of information are found in other countries. In Italy, Roman Catholic organizations are introducing local pre-retirement programs. In Australia, Councils on the Aged have pilot programs. In the United Kingdom, pre-retirement courses and counseling are offered by some employers, voluntary associations, and educational institutes. Orientation also comes in the UK from mutual support groups in churches and local communities. There is a Pre-Retirement Association to advise employers and help organize courses.

The year 2000

Taking comments from various countries at a glance, it appears that little is expected to be done systematically by the year 2000. However, awareness of the need for retirement education will grow. As the UK respondents put it, problems will be the same but more widely recognized. Experts in Nigeria, Egypt, India, Philippines, Kenya, Australia, and US are more or less agreed on this assessment.

The Italian view is that people will be better prepared for the retirement years in 2000, but this will involve opportunity for paid employment to supplement pensions. In the Federal Republic of Germany, the experts there say, heightened awareness will produce improved preparations. The Polish perspective is that the popularization of gerontology will produce interest in post-retirement activities, but preparatory measures will be inadequate.

Only Israel clearly foresees widespread pre-retirement programs, stemming from greater employer participation. By contrast, in Brazil, where serious unemployment is expected to prevail, pre-retirement preparations based on working seem far-fetched.

Recommendations

An expert's consensus is evident for lifelong education in coping with retirement and other "life transitions". Presumably, this education would be pursued in schools and work-places. This recommendation is shared by experts from nations with economies as different as the United States and Nigeria. Particularly important to American observers is the development of new kinds of jobs for middle-aged adults who wish to change career paths. Such jobs could be provided through a proposed National Corps of Youth and Aging, the US experts say; such a proposed vehicle would help to conciliate intergenerational interests.

A frequent recommendation is for a blending of employment and retirement. This could be accomplished in two ways. First, workers could sample retirement, at least in the sense of exploring recreational and leisure interests, by gradual reduction of the time spent in paid employment after age 40 or 50. The reduction could be accomplished by working fewer hours in the day, fewer days in the week, and fewer weeks in the year.

A second, but not necessarily a substitutive, approach would be flexible retirement. The individual, upon reaching conventional retirement age, would have the option to continue working but at reduced hours, in an advisory or supplementary role in the same line of work, or in another capacity making suitable use of his or her talents and perhaps requiring re-training.

The use of the work-place as a major site for retirement education also is widely suggested. Employers would institute educational courses during or after working hours. However, at least in Australia, employers appear reluctant to make time available.

To carry out systematic retirement preparation, the experts point out that counselors and lecturers would have to be trained and materials developed. Who would finance the training and materials? What would the content be? Who would have basic responsibility for developing a systematic approach?

Experts from different countries give different answers. The Japanese experts suggest that retirement courses should be prepared by experts and then adapted by local participants for their own needs. They propose that retirees be brought into the orientation programs that major companies offer young recruits. The retirees could relate their experiences as employees and their reactions to retirement. Not only might retiree participation induce recruits to adjust their own career plans and to make retirement preparations, but retiree participation might also stimulate the elders to plan for their own futures.

At about age 40, in the view of West German observers, employees should be oriented toward the personal issues of getting old. This, rather than a purely retirement focus, should animate programs given on company time. Several companies, they suggest, might pool resources to make programs available to the workers. Social gerontologists should be available to advise families about problems of old age.

The Italians think courses to prepare people just before retirement are useless. Rather, people should be oriented early in life toward enjoying leisure and avoiding over-concentration on a work career. Work should be made pleasant and spread through more of the lifespan. Pensions should be available routinely to anyone too disabled to earn a living.

Measures of promoting good health throughout life should be part of retirement preparation, the Swedish experts say. They would like programs to cover avoidance of excessive alcohol and tobacco use, acceptance of dietary and physical exercise regimens, and promotion of safety measures for dangerous occupational and leisure activities (or abandonment of these activities). The contribution of lifestyle to deteriorations seen in old age should be emphasized. Aging should be seen as having positive aspects. Instead of attempting to deny their own aging, people should be made aware of the corrosive images they have of later life. The use of cosmetic products to conceal age is evidence of a stigma attached to getting old.

The Polish experts look at preparation for retirement as a concern not only of individual and society, but also of industry and government. Thus, government and industry should be concerned with developing services, adapting housing, and removing architectural barriers. Individual preparation involves acquiring information about processes of aging and diseases of old age, pension systems, and leisure or recreational needs. Society assists through policies for helping the infirm, for countering age prejudice, and for creating economic prosperity supportive of old age.

Indian experts call for comprehensive pre-retirement counseling programs by public and private employers. A good program, they say, should begin at recruitment of the employee, and should cover health education, career planning, and development of skills, as well as housing, income, and social and psychological needs in retirement.

Also emphasizing the theme of lifelong preparation for retirement, the UK experts propose the training of physicians and other health workers in counseling individuals on non-work problems, including marital problems. Retirement would be less of a shock if people balanced work and leisure throughout their lives and if employers encouraged such an attitude.

Similarly, the Australians believe that retirement is too narrow a focus. The approach should be propagated by the mass media, and by community, occupational, and other agencies. Rather than limiting orientation efforts to the period just before retirement, personnel departments of businesses should encourage earlier life activities that enrich the individual spiritually, intellectually, and physically.

Likewise, the Nigerians would use the educational and work systems for disseminating information on retirement life and needs, and the Filipino experts propose that employers assist pre-retirees with courses on life management, as well as by helping them with re-training to develop skills suitable for later-life employment.

The Brazilian concern is for maintaining income so that retirement does not mean poverty. This objective justifies laws against age discrimination in employment, as well as guaranteed employment, professional guidance and job placement, re-training so older workers can keep up with new technological demands, fair wages, and good working environments. Retirees should have the option of working part-time without loss of social insurance benefits. Individuals who cannot find employment in the pre-retirement years should receive support until eligible for a pension.

The only experts recommending that retirement preparation be a mandatory component of collective bargaining agreements are the Israelis. They call for laws to support adult education to meet the needs of retirees and pre-retirees. Programs should be initiated several years before retirement so that employees may acquire or deepen good habits of leisure, recreation, and continuing education. Such programs should be devised by employers and unions in consultation with gerontologists and associations of the aged.

Chapter 11
ASSURING RETIREMENT INCOME

Order of priority given to "Income":

1	EGYPT	INDIA	PHILIPPINES	UK	USA
2	AUSTRALIA	ISRAEL	ITALY		
3	BRAZIL	POLAND			
4	JAPAN				
5	W GERMANY				
6					
7	KENYA				
8	FRANCE	NIGERIA			
9	SWEDEN				

The main problems today

Major avenues to assured income in old age are: paid employment, old-age pension, and earnings-related private pension or social
insurance benefit.

Adequacy of income depends on how well it covers the goods
and services the elderly person must buy. Where housing, social
services, and health services are subsidized, the cash income requirement is obviously less. Health status also may be a factor in determining adequacy of retirement income when services must be bought
out of pocket.

Adequacy of income also depends on the status of a nation's
economy. In the less developed world, retirement – in the sense of
completing a span of years at work during which entitlement has
been established to retirement benefits – may be a novelty. Most
rural Indians experience nothing like retirement in the Western sense.
In urban India, inadequate retirement income is the rule. In Nigeria,
people generally are poor, if not destitute, for their entire lives. Kenya
lacks even a rudimentary national system of income and service
supports in old age.

In more developed countries, pension systems may provide little
income for workers and leave widows and surviving dependent

children without coverage. Little is done to prevent old-age poverty due to early retirement when the system offers a benefit actuarially reduced from an inadequate level. Ironically, some systems allow women, who have longer life expectancy, to retire with full benefits at an earlier age than men. However, women generally have not been in the paid work-force long enough to be eligible for maximum benefits.

Inadequacies are all the more ominous because incentive for discretionary saving is almost nil in inflationary times.

Adding to these general statements are the experts' specific observations on problems in their own countries.

Many elderly persons emigrated to Israel so late in life that they lack coverage by a work-related pension. Some cashed in their pension rights in exchange for lump-sum severance pay when they switched jobs, exposing their surviving dependents to risk of poverty. Many immigrants to Israel have only a small state pension.

In Australia, high rents and inflation erode savings and investments. The elderly can fall back on pensions, some of which are indexed to prices, but these provide for only a minimal standard of living, certainly one much lower than pre-retirement income.

In Italy, trade union emphasis on the highest take-home pay for workers means that relatively little is left for pensions. The pension system, described as chaotic, is about to be reformed.

In many countries, retirement benefits are fully or partially indexed for inflation. In Poland, where income dwindles upon retirement, pensions are not indexed; consequently, living standards for retirees are poor and deteriorate. They lack savings.

The pension picture in West Germany is mixed. Some pensions are inadequate. Because they consider public assistance to be charity, many potential claimants forego asking for it. Other pensioners live handsomely in retirement, with about two-thirds of their recent gross salary replaced; but, say the experts, this is not an entirely happy situation, because it encourages or forces retirement of some people and precludes general improvements in health and unemployment insurance. In addition, women's work-related pensions are inadequate owing to past exclusions from gainful employment. The tax rate of a wife working part-time is considered heavy. For all retirees, the costs of energy erode their living standards.

Concern about extremes of income in retirement is expressed in the United Kingdom. Many professionals and executives who lived well during their working careers do far better than many individuals still in the work force. Inflation takes its toll of savings and non-indexed pension income. Pride and ignorance of benefit possibilities deter many elderly persons from seeking aid through means-tested programs.

Similar concern about income extremes is cited by the French. Particularly hard hit are retirees with just enough resources to be ineligible for social help. Worst off are widows and 2–3 million elders entitled only to a minimum pension.

Even in the United States, although about 15 % of the elderly are in "official poverty"– a stringent standard – an additional 15–20 % of the elderly may be considered to be in poverty. With inflation eroding the dollar, improvement in governmental and private income-maintenance programs is difficult to achieve. In a sense, the American goal of adequate retirement income based on savings, private pension, and social insurance remains to be fully realized, because the tripartite elements individually are weak. At the same time, early-retirement options are seen as jeopardizing the possibility of improvement, and the social security system is under attack as being on the brink of bankruptcy.

Sweden offers the example of relatively small disparity between worker and retiree income. Poverty among the elderly is minimal, but Swedish experts see difficulties in maintaining this favorable situation in the face of slow national economic growth and demands of workers for keeping their living standards intact despite inflation. Inter-generational hostility may deepen in the stagnant economy.

Policies and programs today

All the surveyed countries have some programs for providing income in old age. But these programs often do not assure what the experts would consider an adequate living standard.

The governmental programs range from non-contributory old-age pensions to contributory social insurance benefits. Payments may be in lump sums upon retirement, monthly payments whether retired or not, and means-tested allowances. Most countries provide for widows and children of a deceased beneficiary.

Private pension systems on a large scale appear in the more developed countries. Government workers and others in specific occupations may be covered even in countries that lack a well-developed system for workers in general.

In many countries, there are organized efforts to provide reduced-rate or subsidized services in transportation, recreation, cultural events, and education in addition to housing, health, and social care. Almost all countries provide some form of health insurance or service for the elderly.

Most countries provide for full or partial indexing of benefits to wage or price levels. This is done as a means of protecting the elderly from diminished purchasing power during periods of heavy inflation, as well as to improve their living standards as national productivity rises.

By and large, in the more developed countries, governmental programs permit payment of pension at age 60 or 65. In some countries, the individual need not be retired to receive an old-age pension from the State. However, earnings-related pensions may be contingent on retirement.

Lump sum payments are more likely found in less developed nations. Theoretically, they allow the recipient to make an investment or purchase an annuity or go into a small business. The poor individual who exhausts the lump sum may find, in countries like India and Egypt, that no sizeable supports are available other than charity.

Several more-developed countries employ a tiered approach to assuring income in old age. For example, in Sweden, everyone is entitled to an old-age pension whether retired or not after age 65. Workers may increase the benefit by delaying the start of payments until later ages. Besides the universal pension, everyone aged 65 is entitled to a full earnings-related pension (or a reduced pension between ages 60 and 65). The amount of this pension is a proportion of the difference between average annual covered earnings and the universal pension. Individuals without an earnings-related pension receive a larger universal pension.

Other patterns are found: France has social insurance plus mandatory private pension systems; the United States has social insurance, governmental supplements to the poor, and private pensions; Japan has dual social insurance – employees' pension insurance, with provision for contracting out of the government program for one privately administered, and a national pension program for persons excluded from any other program; Israel has public and private pension systems, including a flat-rate and a means-tested supplemental program; and Australia has an old-age pension, means-tested to age 70, with pensioners entitled to subsidized housing.

The year 2000

Looking at the future, the experts seem to wonder if government programs will be able to keep up with commitments. Australia's comments represent major worries about inflation (it may degrade living standards in general), the capacity of voluntary organizations to aid the elderly, unemployment (that is, shrinking opportunities for supplementary retirement income), and further trends to earlier retirement (straining the tax system and individual resources).

Basic to these concerns is fear that economies will stagnate, or grow much more slowly than in the past, leaving little to improve pension systems, if not eroding their foundations.

Paraphrased, here are some comments about the future:

Brazil: Unemployment rates, now high even among those in their mid-30s, won't diminish; there will be an alarming increase in the number of destitute elderly. Brazil needs a million new jobs a year and directed development in poverty-stricken areas.

Egypt: The burdens of pensions and social security will rise as the number of elderly increases and inflation aggravates financing of benefits.

India: Because of inflation, retirees will have inadequate income and workers will have trouble saving for retirement.

Italy: Present problems will worsen, necessitating basic reforms.

Japan: Future workers may be unable to handle the rising burden of supporting the elderly.

UK: Because of rising numbers of elderly, problems will worsen. Political strains may occur if the elderly fashion themselves into a credible political force; if they do not, their share of national wealth will be low.

Sweden: Paying off foreign debts will dog the next generation of workers, simultaneously confronted by swelling ranks of elderly and their pension needs.

US: Inflation will continue and produce a major social-security crisis in the 1980s, even though it is not providing adequate support. The elderly may be scapegoats for economic frustrations as their needs consume proportionately more of the federal budget, perhaps 40% by the year 2000.

Israel: As more and more retirees qualify for a full pension, retirement incomes will rise. Pension plans may have trouble in balancing resources and commitments, especially if inflation continues, population growth and labor-force participation diminish, and life expectancy rises.

Poland: Retirement income will improve in general, but landless retired farmers will lack assistance.

138

West Germany: The prospects for improving pensions are unclear, because total economic development is unclear. However, workers will have more elderly persons to support and there will be demands to rationalize conflicting income-maintenance systems.

Nigeria: The gap between rich and poor will widen, and modernization will bring the kinds of problems that exist in developed nations.

Philippines: Chances of re-employment for the elderly will diminish because they will lack skills and re-training opportunities.

Kenya: Growth of the elderly population will create pressure to resolve issues of their sharing in the expected rise in living standards.

Recommendations

There are numerous proposals for assuring adequate income in the retirement years. They fall into several categories:

1. The national economy

Expand the national economy so that resources are available to make pension and social insurance programs secure and more widespread.

2. Pension and social insurance

Assure the actuarial soundness of pension and social insurance programs by such methods as:

(a) raising the eligibility age,

(b) raising contribution rates.

Assure that everyone has enough income for at least a decent living standard:

(a) reform or expand systems to cover widows and survivors,

(b) institute means tests or other methods for focusing governmental programs on those most in need of support,

(c) make jobs available so that older persons can add to pension and social-insurance income,

(d) index pensions and social insurance to price or wage levels, in order to compensate for inflation.

139

Rationalize or coordinate the mix of public and private programs, so that nobody is over- or under-supported in retirement.

3. Individual efforts

Make jobs available so that older persons can supplement pension, social insurance, and savings.

Channel industrial development to favor creation or maintenance of labor-intensive jobs, to balance the increased mechanization that tends to reduce job opportunities for the elderly.

Promote savings among workers and educate them to provide better for their old age.

Establish gainful activities – for example in handicrafts, cottage industries, and small businesses – in which the elderly can utilize their skills and abilities.

As evident elsewhere in the Sandoz Institute survey, the more developed and the less developed countries share certain concerns and are divided on others. In countries lacking mature social insurance and pension programs, proposals focus on improving them. In one instance, the experts seem to ignore collective actions and focus on individual efforts. The Indian focus is on inculcating the importance of savings among low-income workers, including agricultural laborers, and on organizing savings plans for workers in small-scale enterprises in the so-called unorganized sector (250 million people).

More often, however, the less developed nations seem to emphasize improvements in social insurance and pension programs and in the national economy, so that jobs are created. Egypt is very much concerned about raising gross national product, and doing so in a way that helps preserve traditional community supports for the elderly; for example, home crafts should be encouraged. At the same time, the Egyptian commentators would like to see the young encouraged to take up agriculture, thus preserving community life.

Similarly, Nigeria looks to comprehensive, integrated community development. The Nigerian experts suggest the use of organized age peers, found in some ethnic groups, as sponsors and promoters of such projects as building schools, dispensaries, community centers, and old people's homes, which would provide employment opportunities for retirees. The Philippines emphasizes labor-intensive and cottage industries, and handicrafts.

For Kenya, the main issues are developing social insurance systems and creating part-time jobs for the elderly. Brazil also presses for collective and individual efforts: the adoption by government of social and economic programs benefiting the elderly specifically, as well as policies of national economic growth and reduction of age discrimination in employment.

Actuarial soundness of pension systems, and their rationalization in the interests of efficient use of resources, are concerns of Israel and Italy. Israeli commentators propose integrating national insurance pensions with work-related pensions. When fully operative, these systems – if uncoordinated – would replace 86–100% of earnings, considered exceptionally high. Some experts think 60–70% would be desirable. Through integration, support levels could be reduced, both systems could be stabilized, and the potential disincentive to work could be removed. For Italy, the proposal is to scrap the present pension mix and ultimately to establish a guaranteed minimum income for everyone.

Assuring actuarial soundness requires methods of lengthening the span of working life over which contributions are made, and reducing the number of years in retirement over which benefits are paid out. Both results can be obtained by delaying retirement. The Israeli response suggests development of financial incentives for keeping people at work, such as offering larger pensions for deferral of retirement, reducing the income tax for people who continue to work after reaching retirement age, and subsidizing employers who hire older workers.

The Australian accent is on abolishing pensions that are free of income tests and on encouraging individual savings, particularly through the purchase of indexed annuities under employer-employee arrangements. (Such annuities would maintain purchasing power despite inflation.) The Australians propose raising the eligibility age to 65 (from 60) for women's old-age pensions and granting lump-sum retirement payments in a way that encourages pensions in instalments. Also called for is a policy of guaranteed minimum income, financial planning and counseling for the aged, the indexing of all retirement benefits, and incentives for small businesses involving the elderly.

High on the West German list of proposals are reversing the trend to lower retirement ages, strengthening old-age pensions, and eliminating the earnings related pension. Britain is concerned with narrowing pension differentials through taxation, thereby permitting an increase of pensions for those who had the lowest earnings. Raising British pensions to the West European average and indexing them for inflation are proposed.

Foreseeing major reductions in living standards for pensioners and workers, the Swedish experts ask for a policy that protects the weakest groups (such as the chronically ill) from losses in benefits. No major change in the structure of income supports is proposed.

The American experts, considering their social security system outmoded as well as financially unbalanced, propose its replacement with an income-tested program guaranteeing a minimum annual income, financed from general revenues rather than an earmarked payroll tax. The experts maintain that the costs of such a program might be more than offset by "savings" through withdrawal of benefits from wealthy and moderately well-off individuals.

Chapter 12

RETIREMENT POLICIES

Order of priority given to "Retirement":

1	JAPAN					
2						
3	PHILIPPINES					
4						
5						
6	EGYPT	FRANCE				
7	W GERMANY	INDIA	POLAND	USA		
8	SWEDEN	UK				
9	AUSTRALIA	BRAZIL	ISRAEL	ITALY	KENYA	NIGERIA

The main problems today

The experts' discussion of retirement policies is cast largely as a discussion of work exclusion.

In many countries, retirement is considered a euphemism for chronic unemployment, a result of pressure to transfer jobs to younger workers. Retirement also is considered as an escape from boring, unsatisfying, and unsafe jobs, and as a necessity to claim benefits when adequate support for disability is lacking. At the same time, there is growing recognition that retirement can produce economic deprivation, if not poverty, loss of social and self-esteem, and physical and mental illness.

Retirement is not experienced as an option but as an obligation, say the French experts. Therefore, they continue, it is experienced as a form of exclusion. Pensioners are deprived of a right to work.

It is plain that retirement, all over the world, is rarely perceived as a positive event by the experts. The American, Kenyan, and Israeli observers are alone in explicitly identifying as a problem the widespread failure to conceive of the retired individual as a socially valuable resource. Experienced older workers can enhance the quality of a nation's output, say the Israelis.

Problems stem from the use of retirement to solve job shortages,

143

by decreasing the retirement age as unemployment grows, say the West German experts. Thus, retirement comes too soon or too suddenly for many individuals and they have trouble coping with the loss of a work role and the adoption of a replacement. The Americans also list pressures to retire as a main problem. These include pressures from the employer and society at large.

The individual who chooses to retire, or is in effect forced to retire, may discover boredom in retirement because he or she never developed any leisure interests outside the job, say the Americans, French, Brazilians, and others.

Experts of most countries identify inadequate retirement income as a leading problem and contributant to post-retirement shock. In Italian eyes, pensions fail to support a decent living standard. The Australians note that increasing longevity poses funding problems for pension plans. The Egyptians find that compulsory retirement at age 60 often triggers health and psychological problems, thus creating sickness expenses for families and society.

Despite these negative aspects, the experts in many countries see trends toward earlier retirement. In Australia, such a trend may be influenced by the levels of pension available at particular ages. In Sweden, where an individual may elect a pension between the ages of 60 and 70, there is an ever-decreasing number of persons actually working. The freedom to choose one's pensioning age is, in reality, limited in regions where unemployment is high and suitable work is scarce. Recently early retirement was made less attractive.

Some proposals for raising the age at which full social security benefits become available have been advanced in the US, which happens to be one of the few countries with a law against age discrimination in employment. Federal jobs have no age ceiling; private sector employees are prohibited generally from setting an age lower than 70.

Although women have a longer average lifespan than men, women often may retire on a pension earlier than men. For example, the retirement age for women is 60 in Poland, Brazil, and Israel, versus 65 for men. West Germany also cites earlier retirement for women as a problem.

Public sector workers are required by law to retire at certain ages in Australia, the Philippines, and Brazil. Whether mandated or not, retirement at fixed ages is considered a problem that might be alleviated if rational criteria based on job performance could be devised and accepted. As the American response puts it, retirement based on age is increasingly recognized as a deficient substitute for retirement based on scientifically determined criteria of job performance. Currently, however, such assessments are based on inappropriate criteria – that is, criteria of physical ability suited to young people or not truly reflecting requirements of the job.

In a statement mirroring a dilemma, the Egyptian experts point out that compulsory retirement at age 60 often produces sickness, but raising the retirement age will promote unemployment in younger groups unless the number of jobs increases. In India, job-based medical benefits are lost upon retirement from the organized sector of the economy, thus exposing the retiree's limited resources to rapid depletion if professional care is sought for serious illness.

Policies and programs today

Some type of pension or social insurance program exists in the 16 surveyed countries. The degree of coverage and adequacy of cash benefit varies considerably. Other retirement benefits may include medical and hospital services, housing privileges, tax breaks, investment counseling, and concessions on transportation, recreation, and educational fees.

In some countries, major income-maintenance programs are coordinated to some degree; in others, they are not. For example, Australian experts say that programs in the public and private sector are uncoordinated and vary in quality. The government has no apparent intention to produce a consistent policy for all sectors. In Italy, by contrast, pension reform is contemplated, with provision against an individual's holding multiple pensions.

In India, access to a pension plan varies. Worst off are agricultural workers. Comprising most of the labor force, they do not even have coverage by provident funds (to which employers and employees contribute) or gratuity funds (no employee contribution).

Age of retirement often is stipulated in collective bargaining agreements in many countries. Early retirement may be an option. Most pension arrangements in the UK offer little flexibility. As noted, the US has a law prohibiting discrimination in employment because of age.

In some countries, tentative steps toward phased and flexible retirement are being taken. An Israeli survey showed that about three in four companies have a flexible retirement rule. Of these, two-thirds allow workers to keep their jobs after the usual retirement age is reached, one-quarter permit the retiree to be re-employed in some other job, and one-tenth decide according to need. Professionals have the greatest flexibility in staying on in their jobs in Israel. In

Poland, half-time employment may be arranged in occupations where there is a labor shortage.

In many countries, an early pension is granted for health reasons in public or private systems. Early retirement also may be encouraged to make room for younger workers, or to retain the young when reducing payrolls.

The year 2000

Predictions tend to be dire – inter-generational conflicts over jobs (West Germany), growing class differences based on who is excluded (Sweden), inability to maintain retirement funds (Australia), continued lack of retirement preparation (Brazil), more years in unemployment as life expectancy rises (Egypt), and deepening poverty because of inflation (India).

A few optimistic notes are sounded. Nigeria foresees more people in pension-covered work, though the bulk of the population still will lack coverage. More people will have pensions in Italy.

Recommendations

A basic recommendation from experts in Sweden, the US, and other more developed countries is for more savings during the working years. The US experts propose that unions negotiate for increased private pension benefits in lieu of current wage increases. The Swedish view is that the elderly will benefit from full employment, which requires investment in productive capacity. Immediate consumption must be sacrificed to achieve investment and full employment, the Swedes say. They propose development of capital foundations owned and controlled by employees.

Another basic recommendation is for flexible and phased retirement. Creation of advisory and other positions for older workers is suggested by the Japanese experts. The Australians recommend alternatives to full employment in the form of consulting, advisory, and teaching roles for the elderly. Private employers, aided by government subsidies, should hire and re-train marginal workers, say the US experts.

The Australians emphasize that pension rights should be vested and made portable through statute, and that provision should be made to ensure that retirement funds are operated truly in contributors' interests.

Poland, West Germany, Israel, and Nigeria highlight a need for objective, functional criteria for determining when to retire. Ability and desire to continue at a job, not age, should be considered in designing programs of flexible retirement, the Israelis say. The West Germans want social policy on age of retirement to be based on different life expectancies by gender, and on economic, medical, psychological, and social considerations.

From the UK comes the suggestion for gradual transition to retirement by reducing hours of work between ages 40 and 60, with income deficit made up by the state pension scheme. The Japanese call for availability of part-time and volunteer work for elders. The Americans propose that older workers have an opportunity for education and re-training, in order to make delayed retirement attractive to them and employers.

The Italians want retirement needs and opportunities to be considered in a broad context, and call for parliamentary discussion of pension needs along with employment, income, production, and social security goals for the country. Pensions based on earnings and pensions to meet basic living needs should be differentiated, with the latter reserved for those in dire need.

The Australians would like retirement "villages" to promote social, cultural, recreational, and occupational challenges, in the belief that these promote well-being.

ROUND TWO

ROUND TWO

Introduction

Round two of the Sandoz Institute study was devoted to questions related to the process of making policy for the expanding populations of elderly persons around the world:

1. The elderly, defined as those aged 60 and above, are a highly diverse group. To what extent should they form a target for social policy as a group, and how should their diversity be taken into account by policy-makers?

2. What are the future prospects of jobs being available for the elderly?

3. What is the political context of policy-making for the elderly, in terms of their representation in politics by themselves and others?

4. To what extent can research be of value in policy-making, or in changing public opinion or understanding about problems of the elderly?

5. Finally, the experts were asked for the messages they would most like to communicate to policy-makers.

Chapter 1

DIVERSITY AND POLICY-MAKING

"At no other stage in life are the differences between individuals more marked than in old age," comment the West German experts. Differences are apparent in physical and mental health, income, social status, and ability to meet both day-to-day and dramatic challenges of later life.

Attaining the age of 60, 65, or older does not in itself create a condition meriting special treatment. Nonetheless, the experts generally have grounds for justifying special attention to the elderly population. They note that society has segregated the elderly through exclusion from work and other meaningful roles on the basis of age — a dubious criterion of ability to function in work, family, and community roles.

The elderly have problems like those of younger people, but these problems tend to pile up and become overwhelming. Compound losses within a short period of time undermine autonomy and self-confidence. They include losses of social and economic roles, income, family supports as members die, and health. Health problems tend to be multiple and chronic.

The experts recognize that diversity and commonality of needs must be balanced. But they tend to differ on how to strike the balance for policy-making in their own national contexts.

For example, the West German experts see hardly any good arguments for gearing policy to the elderly as a category, except that general policies fail to meet the needs of the elderly, as in housing. The West German experts fear that measures designed specifically for the aged may encourage a negative image of them. Overall, the best policy is to enable the elderly to decide for themselves the kinds and quantity of help they need, rather than to distribute resources among them according to a fixed system. In practical terms, this means that the elderly must have enough income to buy what they need, a large range of options, and information on which to base choices. The West German experts add that the range of options should cover such activities as early retirement, work in the retirement years, plurality and competition in services, and various housing arrangements.

To the Israelis, major problems of the elderly are universal – such as financial security, family and social support, and health needs. "The elderly differ (from younger adults) only in that they experience these problems with greater intensity. It is this greater intensity that warrants special policy consideration," the experts say. However, the Israelis advise policy-makers that intensity of need varies among the elders and therefore flexibility is required in programs. Some programs should apply to all, such as adequate pensions. Other programs should apply only to those who need the specific benefits, they add.

Experts from within one country may differ on the use of age for programming. One US expert says the elderly are a separate group, because of losses and needs. It is better to deal with them as an age group in making policy than to deal according to disability or other category. At the same time, this expert would have diversity recognized by using various age thresholds as eligibility criteria for different programs: starting in the early seventies for social programs and in the mid seventies for health programs. Diversity of individual patterns of needs should be recognized through such methods as case management, with monitoring to discourage any over-use of benefits at the instigation of providers of services.

A second US expert believes that public policy should be targeted to particular categories of older adults, especially those in groups with higher risks of dependence. In particular, policy-makers should focus programs on the risks from socio-environmental conditions and lifestyles that could be modified to change the character of old age. (In an aside to policy-makers in the developing nations, the expert advises against counting up the elderly population and treating it as inevitably dependent: to exaggerate problems by not making distinctions will immobilize the policy analyst.)

A third US expert advises against making policy for the elderly as a group. Because the elderly are so diverse, it is hard for them or their patrons or champions to formulate a consensus with any practical, specific programmatic significance. While it may be simpler to base policy on age than to base it on distinctions that are less readily measured, doing so is uneconomical: it does not target resources efficiently on those most in need. Moreover, the expense of giving benefits to those not needing them will stir up inter-generational conflict.

The British experts point out that the elderly have been defined historically on an age basis by retirement programs. A political reason for an age basis is that it produces large numbers. From the viewpoint of providing services, treating this large number as a group enables individuals to pass from one pattern of need to another without having to suffer the trauma of transition from one identity group to another. Professionals and the public appear more accepting of a group with a spectrum of conditions and needs, varying from the fit to the bedridden, than they would of a group characterized by unalloyed dependency.

There are pragmatic grounds for flexibility in programming to take differences into account, although demarcation lines for establishing eligibility may become inappropriate over time and often may become stigmatizing. Nonetheless, difficulties in making policy for diverse categories of the elderly can be overcome. They are trivial obstacles, though the UK experts suspect that they may be exaggerated by people who want to reduce services or facilities for the elderly. The experts suggest that policy-makers pay close attention to the capacity of epidemiology to identify groups in need of specific kinds of support.

Because of diversity among the elderly, policy-makers should endorse a diversity of services, the Australian experts say. If used elastically, the concept of old age divided into a Third Age and a Fourth Age would be useful to policy-makers, according to the UK and other commentators. The Third Age is marked by relative independence, and the Fourth Age by increasing weakness and relative dependence. Some experts would define the Fourth Age roughly as starting in the late 70s or early 80s. (The Japanese would modify this rough guide by gender, to take the shorter life expectancy of men into account.)

An advantage of this dichotomy, say the British, is that it turns policy-makers away from viewing the aged monolithically as "victims" of nature or chance. Rather, policy-makers should see that later life may contain a variety of developments. Thus, social policy is not limited to remedial postures but may be directed toward preventive actions, such as postponing the Fourth Age by measures of preventive medicine, health maintenance, and psychosocial aid.

In the French view, several stages should be considered by policy-makers: (a) the sixties, marked by adapting to retirement and preparation for very old age, (b) the seventies, marked by the advent of disabilities, and (c) the eighties and after, marked by an effort to maintain or restore autonomy. These stages may vary by individual, so that eligibility for benefits tied strictly to age would be unsuitable. The prime policy objective, says one French observer, is to prevent slipping into dependency. A sound policy would be oriented to promotion of social and physical activity for the well elderly. At the same time, facilities and services must be prepared for those who have lost their ability to function independently in the community.

The Japanese, too, distinguish several age categories, each with different challenges for policy-making. According to one Japanese commentator, there are the early elderly, aged 55–64, who need jobs; the middle elderly, aged 65–70, who are still active, have a pension, and can get part-time work; and those aged 70–74, who can rely on a full pension. Those over age 75 tend to need services.

A different point about the need for flexibility of policy is offered by the Italians in terms of changes in the characteristics of successive waves of entrants into old age. The Italian experts urge policy-makers to consider socio-economic trends: more of tomorrow's elderly in Italy will have better education; more will have fuller pensions and higher incomes to rely on. Demography also is emphasized by the Swedish experts. The proportion of elderly persons in Sweden will rise to as much as 22% by the year 2000 and then decline somewhat. However, those aged 85 and older will compose a larger proportion of this slightly declining elderly population. The implication of this variation is that demand for services will be larger than the total number of elders would suggest. For example, the incidence of hip fracture is much higher in the Fourth Age than in the Third Age. By age 75, many Swedish women will have lost their husbands; widowhood and living alone are factors that raise the risk of serious illness.

By and large, the task for policy-makers in the more developed countries may be summed up by a Polish comment: "The diversity is a challenge to policy, not a deterrent."

In the less developed countries, the needs of the elderly are seen somewhat differently, perhaps because retirement and family factors are different from the more developed lands. The Kenyan constitution recognizes that the elderly are going to form an important social group and they must be served in their diversity. In Nigeria, where the elderly constitute 3% of the population, a policy of diversity is based on community action. In the Philippines, the elderly are seen as a diverse population but also one that has shared concerns and that benefits from appearing politically as a large group with common needs.

Indian policy-makers should take into account age, sex, rural-urban and economic disparities, according to experts from that country. The Egyptian commentators focus attention on the need for reinforcing family relationships. Policy on assisting families should take social class into account. For example, middle-class families may need services to maintain their elderly at home and to continue relating to them in institutions. The primary need in lower-class families is income. The Egyptian experts acknowledge that defining the elderly as a group isolates them from the mainstream of society.

But, they add, the elderly must be considered as a group for purposes of pension and services policy. Moreover, defining the elderly as a broad range of ages allows for mixing people of different capacity in programs and institutions, and suggests a policy of having the younger elderly assist the older elderly.

Overall, the experts in the surveyed countries find grounds for policy-making based on retirement age, but argue for flexible programming to recognize diversity of need.

Chapter 2
JOBS AND POLICY PROBLEMS

Separation from gainful employment, the most common reason for making policy specifically for the elderly, has social as well as economic and political implications. The experts generally note a worldwide trend in unemployment as a reflection of technological change, principally the replacement of human labor by machines. At the same time, more young workers are available than economies appear to have jobs for.

While older workers with certain skills stay in the work-force, experts from various countries report continued trends to early retirement. Policies favoring early retirement as a means of shifting jobs to younger workers are seen by the experts as counter-productive. The policies tend (a) to create physical and mental problems that require social expenditures, and (b) to stretch out the years over which pensions must be paid, resulting in reduced installments and higher rates of poverty and dependency.

The employment picture is generally bleak for at least the short term in every country surveyed, except for Japan, assuming the birth rate there will not rise and the rate of economic growth continues. The elderly in their late fifties and early sixties, however, are at a disadvantage, one Japanese expert notes. These individuals lack jobs and adequate income in the years after retirement at age 55 but before pensions start at age 60, while the older elderly have pensions and part-time income. Raising the age of retirement to 65 is proposed as a means of keeping more older workers on the job. Other proposals are for flexible retirement, job sharing, and holiday, night, and relief tours by older workers.

Problems for the elderly and for youth will not be resolved without a thorough overhaul of the entire economy, say the UK experts. In the 1990s, they foresee considerable under-employment because of technological advances and decline in basic industries. Possibly half the adult population, counting retirees and non-working women, may lack paid employment. Programs for youth employment and early retirement are seen as trivial. Solutions may require shorter hours as part of spreading the work, less stigmatizing of those who have no jobs or are employed part-time, and payment arrangements for persons for whom no full-time work exists. All of this presupposes no conventional or nuclear war, the experts say.

The West German observers say that today's unemployment levels would be substantially higher if an early-retirement scheme had not been introduced in 1972–73. Far more workers opted for early retirement than expected, about two-thirds instead of 20–30%. Government, employers, and unions all favor early retirement. Though this may help the economy in one way, it poses a dilemma in pension finance: pensioners oppose cuts in payments, and insurance plans will go under without cuts. The experts say that proposals to keep the elderly at work must be considered wishful thinking at the moment. The same may be said of Poland, where early retirement is a key policy.

France, too, has opted for early retirement as a solution to joblessness, but a French expert says this is an unproven approach. Unemployment, chronic in France and linked to the European situation, may be a result of technological developments and increases in social security contributions.

A triad of high inflation, unemployment, and recession is pictured in Israel. While the immediate prospect is increasing joblessness, to some extent concentrated by geographical area and occupational category, there is room for cautious optimism. Public policy will not tolerate a long period of unemployment, the Israeli experts say, adding that the full utilization of manpower potential is a matter of deliberate policy rather than blind submission to economic trends.

In Sweden as well as other countries, the experts are concerned that policy will be so heavily biased toward work for the young that the elderly will be stranded without jobs. The elderly are virtually ignored. Swedish proposals focus on educating the young for industry needs. They assume that the young have a greater ability to adjust to new conditions than have older workers despite their skill and experience.

Job shortages in the US are expected by one expert to last until the "baby boom" cohort retires, starting about 2020. another US expert is unsure of long-term prospects. Job availability in the year 2000 will reflect economic conditions and types of activity we cannot presume to know precisely today, this US expert says. There is room for optimism in expected trends away from heavy labor and other occupations that are less favorable for the elderly. If they can keep their skills up to date with modern technology, especially in the services, management, and communications sectors of the economy, older workers may have good job possibilities. Women's problems may diminish, as more of them have regular work and occupy jobs covered by private pensions. Educational opportunities, job training, and a broader occupational distribution will benefit future women. "My optimism is about as well grounded as anyone's pessimism," this US expert declares.

A third US expert sees a counter-trend to early retirement in the making, due to (a) a recent law prohibiting job discrimination by age, (b) inflationary pressure on the elderly to find paid work, and (c) a political decision to promote later retirement as a means of taking pressure off government and pension programs.

In Africa, job shortages also are expected to increase. No specific solutions are proposed for the jobless elderly in Nigeria. The Nigerian experts expect the older worker's security to be assured eventually through general economic development. Likewise, promotion of industry in Kenya, with emphasis on rural industrialization, is seen as benefiting the elderly. However, population growth there will outstrip industrial growth.

The same holds for Egypt, where the population will increase by over 50% by the year 2000. Population control has direct implications for well-being in later life, the Egyptian experts indicate. Migration of skilled workers continues. A general effort toward more technical and vocational training, and more adult education, is regarded as helping to ease the manpower situation. Retirees may have a better chance to find jobs through re-training, the experts say, but the retirement age itself will not be raised, out of consideration for young workers.

In India, chronic unemployment is worsening and retirement at even younger ages in the future is expected. Every less developed country is in the same difficulty, say the Philippine experts, because of growing population, urbanization, and technological changes. Consequently, the basic policy thrust has to be to expand the economy. However, these commentators add, development programs by the government should promote community participation, self-reliance, and self-esteem of the elderly.

Chapter 3

POLITICAL CONTEXTS AND POLICY-MAKING

What role will politics play in producing solutions to the problems identified in Round one of the Sandoz Institute study?

This general question was posed to the experts in an attempt to sample the political implications of growing national populations of elders around the world. Of obvious concern to policy-makers is the likelihood that elderly voters will form a block or constituency, and the extent to which political parties, especially in these days of governmental austerity, will act on their behalf.

The experts' responses indicate a spectrum of national differences. These include awareness of the needs of the elderly by themselves and by others; willingness to form political pressure groups; responsiveness of government, political parties, and the private sector to issues and proposals; and the effect of political processes themselves on the expression and resolution of problems. Coloring all these factors are perceptions and expectations about economic trends and the ability and willingness of a national population to share the costs of change equitably.

As the range of variables may suggest, there are hazards in attempting to make national and international generalizations on any of the foregoing considerations. However a few major points emerge from the experts' responses.

1. The rising numbers and proportions of the elderly in various countries have not given birth to a "politics of age" in any of the surveyed countries. There are no political parties comprised solely of the elderly. There are a few aggressive pressure groups of elderly persons, notably the Gray Panthers in the US, and the Senior Citizens Defense Association of Wuppertal, in West Germany. By and large, there are few demonstrations at the polls of "senior power", and the larger the organization of elderly the less likely it will lobby for radical changes.

The basic political fact is that the elderly generally do not characterize their problems as problems of old age, at least not as problems that are open to political remedy. This may reflect (a) a negative image of aging: people do not want to be identified as "old", (b) a view of their particular problems as extensions of problems affecting society generally, and (c) a tendency of the contemporary elderly in many countries to be politically passive about problems they believe to be in the nature of old age.

Awareness of problems peculiar to old age seems to be absent among the elderly in many of the less developed countries. Elsewhere, awareness may produce lip service by major politicians (including elderly politicians) as well as serious activity within political parties.

2. As an actual or potential constituency, the elderly pose fundamental organizational difficulties. We return to the issue of diversity, raised earlier in this survey. Defining the elderly broadly as a group for which policy should be made produces, at least on paper, a large political constituency. This potential requires group consciousness if it is to be realized, and this appears to be relatively rare around the world. The elderly are diverse in political, social, economic, and other characteristics. Only on the most basic issues are the chances for consensus relatively good. Once basic needs for income or services have been met to some degree, it is the defense of the gains rather than their extension that is likely to unify the elderly with any great fervor.

The reasons for this may be understood by considering the disparate outlooks of poor and rich elders, of well and chronically sick elders, of younger and older elders, and of those elders who have work income and those who want but can't find work. Some may be eager for more benefits while others, seemingly acting against their immediate interest, favor austerity in order to protect the income of their children from higher taxes and to maintain a balance in the national economy that promotes dividends, profits, and international trade advantages. In short, lifelong socio-economic outlooks tend to prevail. In the UK, the older population tends to be conservative because women and the rich are the predominant survivors at older ages, and tend to be conservative in outlook. Competition to preserve or enlarge benefits affecting one sector of the older population rather than another may be divisive, or a group which has achieved its gains may be disinterested in improvements for other elderly groups.

3. Sometimes, the problems of the elderly are more quickly and ardently perceived and pursued by individuals and groups who are not elderly. Leadership may be taken by intellectuals, professionals, business groups, scientists, and others who have an interest in research, training, services, and marketing activities directed at the elderly population. For example, providers of services – doctors, social workers, nursing-home owners, hospital administrators, func-

tionaries in volunteer and religious associations – may be deeply concerned with problems of the elderly and governmental policies. These may be narrow or technical policies concerning reimbursement for services, standards of services, barriers to expansion or coordination of benefits, and eligibility criteria. Labor unions may be interested in retirement policies adopted by government because of their effects on the job market or on negotiations for private pension.

These considerations suggest that the formulation of demands made in the name of the elderly may be conditioned by special agendas, an obvious point but one that imposes on the policy-maker in the aging field a high degree of circumspection. This extends to consideration not only of contemporary problems but also of the impact of policy made today on the future elderly. Debate over policy concerning the elderly is colored by the source of advocacy.

4. In many developed countries, the major political parties tend to have similar policies toward the elderly. This collegiality is under economic stress. With austerity the order of the day, hard political choices are made between policies that have been tolerated and those that have deep roots. In general, parties supported by organized labor continue to favor stronger government programs for the elderly, while conservative parties favor more private sector responsibility. Responsiveness to the elderly is tempered by political party history and outlook.

5. In less developed lands, where the elderly popoulation is growing at a much faster pace than in the more developed countries, awareness of problems of the elderly is rudimentary among voters and leaders, who tend to be absorbed in problems affecting the entire population. In Nigeria, for example, the problems of the elderly are seen as those affecting the vast majority of the people. According to the Nigerian experts, "there is no basis as yet for the elderly to become a subject of partisan politics." In Brazil, political parties are said to ignore the elderly population, which is relatively small. No elderly pressure groups exist, but some potential is seen for the evolution of self-help groups as a political force.

In Egypt, faced with overwhelming economic problems, the political structure generally ignores the elderly. Nonetheless, through training programs for professionals and through television programs, government officials are creating some awareness of elderly problems. Kenyan experts see problems of the elderly as relatively unimportant, because of cultural patterns of family support. In India, no political parties or pressure groups champion the elderly, although many politicians are old.

The remainder of this section on politics turns to a few patterns in more developed countries, where awareness of elderly problems exists in political circles. The UK has a National Association of Old Age Pensioners, made up of former union members and participating in a campaign for higher pensions. Israel has a National Organization of Retirees, a confederation supported by the Labor Party and having influence on the regulation of major retirement funds. West Germany has a Federal Congress of the Elder Generation, which has attacked the political parties for being dominated by younger people and for giving only lip service to the aged.

A Polish organization of elders, the Union of Fighters for Freedom and Democracy, is considered influential with policy-makers, while in France the elderly have no political pressure group, being loath to separate themselves from the mainstream of society. The French experts believe that consciousness as a separate group is developing through the mass media, which offer special programs or appeals to the elderly.

In Sweden, pension groups are considered powerful, and the political parties have similar programs favoring the elderly. Pensioners appear to be better off economically than anywhere else in the world. Conflict nonetheless arises between them and workers, because pensions are indexed to inflation and earnings are not, the experts note. Health-care costs have risen dramatically, sharpening a debate over how much pensioners should pay directly for services they receive.

In Japan, the elderly appear to have weak support in politics, since their problems mainly are considered to be for families to resolve. The experts point out that retirees aged 60 and over are defended by such groups as the National Federation of Old Men's Clubs, the National Social Welfare Council, and, occasionally, the Labor Party. But the recent retiree, aged 55–60, occupies a no-man's land in terms of representation.

By contrast, the US has a wealth of elderly representation though its effectiveness may be debated. One group, the American Association of Retired Persons, has 11 million members aged 55 and older. About 100 "aging-based" groups are counted by an American expert. These are groups that depend on the existence of older people as members, as users of their services, as clients of the practitioners who belong to the aging-based organization, and as subjects of scientific study. These organizations exert influence through government officials, whose programs they may help to legitimate. The thrust of the political activity of most aging-based groups is heavily in their own members' occupational and other special interests, one US expert points out.

In the US, both major political parties tend to favor the elderly. Since the parties seek to avoid alienating other large blocks of voters and taxpayers, they tend to offer mild programmatic improvements. Nor do groups representing elderly interests generally seek drastic changes, except for the Gray Panthers. Unlike the mass membership elderly groups, this group has a small membership that unifies on controversial issues.

Generally, elderly groups are more effective in preventing cuts in benefits than in launching new programs. The principal method of influencing American politics on issues of aging is through discussion in public forums, such as the decennial White House Conferences on Aging. The experts see little evidence that aging-based groups change the predispositions of policy-makers in government, although they often claim credit for doing so. Essentially, these groups lobby and practice public relations, emphasizing issues rather than candidates. No clear test of their political effectiveness seems possible, according to the experts.

Only in scattered community elections is there evidence of block voting by the elderly. This occurs in areas where the elderly voters comprise a relatively large part of the electorate and are sensitive to a particular issue, such as more taxation for schools. In such cases, the vote of the elderly might be characterized as the vote of property owners.

To one US expert, the effectiveness of the elderly in politics will depend on their emphasizing a problem-solving approach, rather than an ideology or principle. For example, this expert believes that the principle of universal benefits should give way to a focus on those most in need. Some problems should be differentiated as susceptible to government or private action. Priorities within one sphere or the other should be determined. Some problems of the elderly will slip off the public agenda as a politics of scarcity takes effect. The emphasis will be on efficient spending and effective targeting of programs. "If any solutions are to be found to the problems identified in the first round of the [Sandoz Institute] study," says an American expert, "they will emerge from a confluence of political, economic, and social forces, not from senior power."

Chapter 4
RESEARCH AND POLICY-MAKING NEEDS

Research can be both a tool and a goad to policy-making. It can change the perception of problems and the nature of problems for which policy is needed, can offer options for action, and can evaluate the courses or interventions taken (on the basis of theory or limited evidence) to see if goals and outcomes are achieved as expected.

However, one of the the most important values of research is to discount myths and fallacies. Because of so much negativism about aging and old people, one effect of research is to produce a balancing positivism. It helps clear the way to action.

Experts in almost all the surveyed nations suggest that fallacies about aging must be corrected as a first policy-making step. Myths about aging tend to create a monolithic picture of the elderly population as dependent. Myths may turn policy-making away from the capacities and potentials of elderly persons in leading active, productive lives, from the potential effectiveness of preventive measures applied throughout lifetime in assuring vigor in old age, from the potentials of families in assisting elderly persons to function at home despite disabilities, and from the socio-environmental barriers to achieving these potentials.

In short, fallacies may misdirect or abort policy-making. Conversely, research findings may show where policy-making is necessary and feasible. As information becomes available to the public, it helps to change the climate for policy-making.

Here is how the experts might respond as a group if asked for a concise statement about what research tells us about aging:

Gerontology research tells us that aging processes are not exclusively conditioned by irreversible biological mechanisms proceeding within the individual. Rather, aging represents the interplay of multiple factors, and is heavily influenced by psychosocial (including economic) factors. Thus, political measures can play a major role in modifying many of the negative characteristics ascribed to old age. This can be done by making the most of human development throughout the lifespan; by applying preventive, therapeutic, and rehabilitative measures whenever necessary; and by assisting people in coping, and learning how to cope better, with their problems and stresses.

165

Among reports the experts suggest as important reading for policy-makers is *Old People in Three Industrial Societies*, by Peter Townsend, Ethel Shanas, and Henning Friis. This work, a decade old, indicated that the elderly in the UK, US, and Denmark were not primarily a burden on society and official services. Rather, they were a section of their communities that continued, to a large extent, to make a contribution to itself and the life of the community as a whole. It showed that the family in industrialized societies was alive and well. Moreover, the family was providing the base for reciprocal services, both material and psychic. It helped public bodies to understand that a central issue of aging was not one of how to provide charity, but of how to utilize a major resource, according to the UK experts. "Other research has directed attention to the fact that social values of the wider society determine policy, not just the material condition of the elderly," the UK commentators add.

Research also indicates that conditions once thought to be concomitants of aging are actually diseases whose occurrence is heavily influenced by socio-environmental factors. This point, too, fosters the realization that policy for the elderly is one aspect of policy for the entire community. According to the UK experts, this perspective helps to liberate people from the notion that the elders are a burdensome client group.

The concept of the "modifiability of aging processes", as a US expert puts it, should be pursued as a matter of both science and policy-making. The world experts concur that life expectancy and sickness rates can be improved. More empirical work is needed to understand the reasons for the vast differences in coping behavior and outcome among the elderly of different ages. The fact that morbidity and longevity rates differ by groups within a country, and between countries, has profound implications.

"We do not know what normal aging is like under optimal social conditions," says an American expert. He notes that under optimal conditions certain familiar risk factors would be eliminated, such as poor diet, cigarette smoking, alcohol abuse, sedentary living, and counter-productive ways of coping with stress. All these risk factors, the expert says, are potentially modifiable.

One of the most dogged fallacies is that senile dementia is an inescapable aspect of human aging. But research is showing that this loss of memory, and eventually destruction of personality, is a disease itself. It occurs only in a minority of the aged. It may be a symptom of treatable disease outside the brain, such as drug toxicity and infection. There is hope that senile dementia may be modified, cured, or prevented even in its primary form, just as other diseases are controlled. Indeed, the neurochemical and other brain derangements of individuals suffering from senile dementia are now being identified. The beginnings of effective drug therapy seem to be taking place.

The experts point to a number of findings for consideration by policy-makers:

1. Intellectual function remains remarkably stable into the seventies and eighties. Exploration has just begun into the importance of motivation in maintaining intellectual functioning, and into demonstrations of how training can improve intellectual functioning in older people. An implication of this research is that past observations about loss of intellect with age may represent failure to examine issues of motivation, and the effects of concurrent disease and negative expectation on the performance of the elderly.

2. Opportunity for maintaining social interaction is critical to the healthy behavior of older adults. Old individuals who have been taught to remain involved in social activity, are expected to remain involved, and have the opportunity, do indeed remain involved – and their general well-being appears to be preserved.

3. A chronically ill elderly person who has a son, daughter, or other family member to rely on is much less likely to be institutionalized than an elderly person without family. The more children an elderly individual has the less seem to be the odds of having to live in a nursing home or other institution, according to several studies, notably one by the US government. Given the high costs of institutionalization, especially to governmental programs, these studies have major policy-making implications.

4. Medical care in old age improves survival rates. While sophisticated observers may take such a finding as too obvious for extensive comment, the experts believe that fallacious notions about aging impede the application of proper medical care throughout life, especially in old age. The belief that medical care is largely unavailing for the elderly is another reflection of misconceptions about the nature of aging and of devaluation of the elderly. Indeed, illness accelerates aging. Knowledge exists for treating and preventing major diseases frequent in old age. More is needed. Early diagnosis and treatment of hypertension is given as a proven example of steps taken earlier in life that can avoid or delay stroke and other cardiovascular diseases in later life. The experts believe that hormonal treatment of the menopause may reduce osteoporosis and risk of fractures.

167

The experts also note current efforts to improve knowledge about the elderly.

Better understanding of the nature of the elderly person in responding to trauma, infection, and therapeutic interventions, particularly to drugs and surgery, is being acquired. Some experts note studies indicating poor diagnosis of the elderly by doctors — not only missing diseases that deserve treatment but providing treatment unnecessarily for conditions that are normal age changes, not diseases. Consequently, improved geriatric knowledge and technique have implications for health costs and manpower needs.

Population studies are identifying biological, psychological, and sociological influences on health status of the elderly, who, in the past, often were ignored even in broad surveys. In particular, probably for the first time, the true epidemiology of senile dementia is being established. A World Health Organization study of urban living conditions of the elderly and their health status, considered a valuable reference for policy-making, should be supplemented by additional investigations. Studies are needed of old people who live alone, and the social and medical factors that affect their lives.

Another valuable type of investigation, longitudinal research, helps to sort out intrinsic and extrinsic changes that seem to occur with age. Many past studies of aging depended on comparing older and younger individuals. These cross-sectional studies were valuable, but open to question as to the extent to which differences in performance represented age differences or differences in personal and social history. For example, conclusions about the inferior ability of elderly individuals in certain intellectual tests requiring pencil and paper may not take into account that they grew up at a time when public education was not as developed as it is today. Performance represented unfamiliarity or unease with testing procedures.

In longitudinal studies, the same individuals are tested periodically over many years according to standardized procedures. This makes it possible to compare the older person to his or her younger self. Many objections to cross-sectional conclusions can be avoided. The longitudinal data also make possible greater precision in determining precursors of later disorders. Such studies may prove invaluable in establishing the earliest indications of senile dementia and cardiovascular malfunction, and provide perspectives on the influence of psychosocial as well as biological factors in "successful" aging.

Intervention studies form a class of research of particular value to policy-making. An eight-year intervention study has begun in Göteborg, Sweden, to determine the extent to which certain socio-environmental changes contribute to improved quality and length of life of people now in their seventies. Being tested is the hypothesis that physical and intellectual activity promotes the well-being of older people. Longitudinal measurements are being made of muscle strength, bone density, heart function, intellectual function, life satisfaction, and social interaction. The costs of the interventions – which include removing architectural barriers and providing regular medical check-ups and occupational services – will be weighed against the benefits and their value. The Swedish experts note that previous Göteborg studies have contributed to policy-making concerning medical care, traffic, housing, and education for the elderly.

The extent to which research conducted in industrialized countries is relevant to the less developed countries is questioned by Nigerian experts. While much of this gerontological research is of value, the experts say that Nigerian policy-making has special research needs. For example, because of the central role of families, research might be directed toward the development of programs of comprehensive family care rather than age-categorical programs of care for just mothers and infants, just children, and just youths. The Egyptians point to special needs to study the effects of endemic diseases on the rural elderly, to find ways of preventing such diseases as schistosomiasis. They also suggest a need for studying the effect on the institutionalized elderly of community roles created for them.

Before less developed nations elaborate institutional structures for taking care of the chronically ill elderly, and before they elaborate social service networks, the countries might well consider a variety of strategies focusing on the family and kinship networks, says a US expert. In a sense, the expert is urging that costly but questionable experiences of the more developed countries might be avoided and valuable resources conserved.

A theme of learning from one another's laboratory, clinical, population, and intervention studies is apparent in the experts' comments. Asked to indicate a few priority areas for policy-oriented research in the future, the experts offered a wide spectrum of suggestions, notably:

1. *On living arrangements*

(a) Evaluate the design of homes, furniture, and access to buildings in terms of enabling older people to live independently in the community for as long as possible.

(b) Study choices the elderly make and would wish to be able to make concerning living arrangement, especially living with or separately from adult children.

169

(c) Experiment with housing and socio-environmental manipulat-ions, rather than narrowly with health-care approaches, in meeting needs for living in the community despite sickness and disabilities.

2. On health care

(a) Conduct studies leading to improved efficacy and efficiency of home-care teams.

(b) Investigate the organization, costs, and effectiveness of various strategies of long-term care based on residence at home or in institutions.

(c) Study methods of preserving and improving the psychosocial and physical functioning of the institutionalized elderly.

(d) Conduct systematic research useful in establishing comprehen-sive long-term care strategies, including: methods of identify-ing individuals who are, and will be, at risk of problems requiring long-term care; methods of assessing patient needs so that services may be directed effectively and efficiently; and methods of predicting the patterns of care most likely to produce improvement, or stem deterioration, with the least undesirable disruption of life style.

(e) Conduct more experiments with alternate modes of meeting long-term care needs.

(f) Develop a basis for evaluating programs of care according to outcome and relative cost.

3. On activity useful to individual and society

(a) Conduct studies on the use of the elderly as a social resource.

(b) Investigate the work capacities of older workers, possible methods of re-training them, and possible adaptations in work arrangements and environments to facilitate their performance and motivation.

4. On patterns of retirement living

(a) Examine how the elderly adapt to retirement, in order to identify patterns of successful and satisfactory adjustment and to de-termine the living conditions preferred by, and most favorable to the well-being of, elderly persons and couples of different ages, backgrounds, and conditions of life.

(b) Survey the elderly on their opinions and wants in the way of public and private services and products.

(c) Study the effects of retirement life on physical and mental activity, and compare the effects of phased and flexible retirement.

5. *On income maintenance*

(a) Examine the effects of current income-maintenance arrangements on the most disadvantaged elderly, including widows and members of ethnic minorities.

(b) Determine the possible effects of mechanisms for integrating public and private pension benefits, so as to assist in developing policies for ensuring that at least an adequate income is available to all.

6. *On formulating and monitoring the results of policy*

(a) Conduct research to determine whether policies adopted for the elderly actually promote or hamper their well-being.

(b) Acquire periodic demographic information on the elderly in five-year age groups, thus facilitating policy formulation and review according to impact on age groups.

To this list the experts add basic biological and psychosocial research and clinical geriatric research, especially into the causes, diagnosis, treatment, and prevention of senile dementia. The experts characterize this disease as most destructive of the ability of elderly individuals to take care of themselves. They believe it will become even more evident as a cause of dependency as cardiovascular diseases, cancer, and other major health problems come under control. Depression, whose causes lie within and outside the individual, especially in the context of later-life socio-economic and health losses, deserves a research priority from a policy-making point of view for much the same reasons as senile dementia: prevention of depression is important to preserving independence.

As policy-makers look more and more to assisting the family to assist the elderly, the experts would urge more research on the changing nature of the family as a group, and on those members on whom responsibility for providing care will fall, particularly on middle-aged women. The evaluation of program impact on these key individuals should be built into policy.

Examination of male-female differentials in need for services and income maintenance is emphasized by some experts.

Finally, the experts call attention to the fact that "aging" is by definition a continuing and universal process of human development. The selection of any particular age to define "elderly" is purely

171

arbitrary. Consequently, some research findings on those aged 75 will point to useful investigations to be made of earlier life patterns. Similarly, scientific findings about early life may have valuable application, or offer valuable insights, to research on later life.

Chapter 5

BEACONS FOR POLICY–MAKERS

As a final question, the experts were asked what single point or brief message they would want policy-makers of their country to consider. Here are the distilled responses:

Australia

Articulate a clear national policy on aging, develop a method for meeting properly assessed needs, and provide national and community programs to meet them comprehensively.

Brazil

Improve the economic condition of the aged so they may feel respected in the community: do this by offering medical and social care, housing, and jobs compatible with physical condition.

Egypt

Make every effort to prevent natural and socio-cultural causes of debilitating stresses, and preserve the extended family.

Federal Republic of Germany

Encourage, early in life, the foundations for activity and well-being in old age by stressing the importance of leisure as well as work activities, and promote policies of flexible retirement.

France

Expert A: Consider elderly persons as *full* citizens, reduce the serious economic inequalities facing them, ensure that elders have equal rights to health care, and prevent their isolation from the rest of society.

Expert B: Develop policy toward the elderly on a life-cycle basis, so different generations perceive their mutuality.

India

Care for the elderly is a national responsibility.

Israel

Base the provision of social services on recognition of the honor and dignity of individuals, as a right, not a philanthropy; support the fulfilment of human potential as part of social justice.

Italy

Expert A: Organize social services in a personalized way to strengthen choice by the elderly person in planning this part of life.

Expert B: Seek to make old age as problem-free as possible, particularly through education and health-care programs.

Japan

Provide options for living with and apart from children, and for working at least to age 70, and provide a respectable living standard.

Kenya

Maintain the extended African family unit.

Nigeria

Bear in mind that aging is continuous from birth and influences, and is influenced by, socio-economic factors.

Philippines

Recognize that aging is a normal phase of human development; include policies for aging people within national policies of social and economic development.

Poland

Expert A: Create feelings of safety and independence, the "water of life" for elderly people.

Expert B: Provide retirement for all the elderly at a decent living standard.

Sweden

Recognize individual differences by offering a variety of retirement options.

UK

Expert A: Change the popular view of retirement as a brief prelude to death, and substitute the view of retirement as the longest period of stability in the lifetime.

Expert B: Recognize that it is in *your* interest to care about aging.

Expert C: Recognize that much age-associated disability is due to socio-environmental factors, rather than intrinsic and inevitable biological ones.

USA

Expert A: Be aware that the country's elderly are vulnerable, they will not go away, and their treatment is a good measure of basic social values.

Expert B: Keep in mind that the elderly are a heterogeneous group, that resources must be targeted on those who need them most, and that, by doing so, leaders will save tax money and reduce inter-generational conflict.

Expert C: Understand that much of what is called "aging" is modifiable, and that hope exists for reducing risks of impairment and dependence.

Economic commentary

In most countries throughout the world, more and more people believe that they are paying too much in taxes and social security contributions. They are being left with too little to spend on themselves. Governments have been responding to this pressure by trying to find ways of cutting public expenditure, or at least curtailing its rate of growth. The most common target for public expenditure cuts has been the "Welfare State" – selected because of its enormous growth as a proportion of public spending since World War II. Not only are the elderly excluded from the mainstream of society, but they are beginning to be blamed for the heavy tax burdens carried by those at work.

Given this world trend, it is perhaps inevitable that the gerontologists and other experts who have participated in the Sandoz Institute survey, covering 16 developed and developing countries, should take a pessimistic view of the prospects for older persons over the next two decades. The elderly add little to the measured gross national product, though many of them may contribute substantially to the care of children and the quality of life of their families in ways which current economic statistics do not measure. Often they make it possible for mothers to take paid work. But what cannot be denied is that, when they receive pensions, the resources these represent have to be found out of the current production of the working population. Pensions represent, in essence, a contract between the generations. Moreover, the elderly have the largest needs for health and social services. Social and medical care for the mentally and physically infirm elderly is costly, whether that cost falls on formal services provided through insurance schemes or tax-financed provisions, or on younger family members – usually women who, as a result, are less able to contribute to measured production. How can we expect our currently over-burdened economies to provide for more elderly, and particularly more very elderly, let alone to improve the standards of what is currently provided? This is the problem facing most societies over the next twenty years.

Overwhelmed as many of us are by gloom about the present, it is easy to get the problem out of perspective and to blame the wrong victims. It is only when we look back at the recent past that the real character and magnitude of the problems which face us in the future fall into place.

177

Lessons from the past

The more developed countries have not come to a sudden point in history when the proportion of elderly has started to increase substantially; the process has been at work throughout this century. Indeed, the rate of growth of the elderly as a proportion of total population is likely to be generally less in the future than it has been in the recent past. The predominant change in prospect for the next two decades is the relatively large growth in the proportion of "old" old (aged 80 and over) as compared with the growth of the total elderly population.

The economies of the more developed countries absorbed the rapid growth of the elderly relatively painlessly in the prosperous 1950s and 1960s. It was in this period that pension schemes, both public and private, were rapidly extended and improved. It was a period also of rapid expansion in spending on health care. Many countries rebuilt most of their hospitals on a new and much more lavish scale, and built accommodation for elderly persons on a more homely scale and with better amenities. In all these ways, old people were given a share of rising prosperity.

But what was different about the fifties and sixties, as compared with the prospect for the eighties and nineties, is that at the same time we were having to provide for the post-Second World War boom in births. We were building homes for couples who were marrying at younger ages. We were building first primary schools, then secondary schools, and finally institutions of higher education. We were training and paying teachers to staff them, and the costs of maintaining children were being shared through family allowances and educational grants.

The double burden of more young and more old did not lead to tax resistance. Indeed, the rapid growth of public expenditure on both age groups was absorbed without protest, because there was still room in our expanding economies for a steady and substantial growth in real take-home pay. Compared with earlier history, the rate of economic growth between 1950 and 1973 was extraordinary.

Now this bulge of the post-war generation has reached working age. It has been more expensively prepared for work than any previous generation. It is equipped to produce the resources out of which planned pensions and better services for the elderly can be financed. As automation reduces the manpower needed to expand industrial production, it is in the service occupations that new jobs can readily be created – particularly for the growing proportion of women seeking paid work. The fall in the birth rate means that there is currently no pressing need to expand education, though there is always room for improving educational standards and for giving wider opportunities for higher education at all ages. Fewer children will be needing family allowances and educational grants. And many countries have built more hospital beds for the acute sick than are really needed, in view of the trend to shorter stays. Much of this excess of social capital can be readily adapted for the use of the elderly chronic sick. In all these respects, the underlying economic problems of demographic change which face the more developed countries are much less daunting than the problems facing them 30 years ago.

The developing countries, on the other hand, continue to be faced with massive competing demands for public expenditure. These will persist whether the economic situation improves or not. Though the developing countries will have a much smaller proportion of elderly in the year 2000 than do the developed countries today, they will still be providing for larger proportions of children and for all the pressing demands of socio-economic development. Only a few have managed to achieve rapid economic growth, although the benefits of this growth have been unequally divided. Nevertheless, these countries are successfully using their lower labor costs to gain an increasing foothold in the world market for the older manufactured goods. This competitive advantage is strengthened by relative lack of development of social security schemes financed in part by employers' contributions, which raise labor costs.

The high proportion of children needs costly education, to prepare them to play their part in the process of development. Only a few countries are clearly on course for the demographic transition to lower birth rates, and even in these countries the size of the school-age population has not yet stabilized.

The cost of the world economic crisis

The fundamental cause of the current gloom is not the demographic prospect but the stagnation of the world economy, triggered by the chronic imbalance in trade between the main oil exporters and the rest of the world. If world trade were still rapidly expanding and the oil surplus were being re-cycled to the developing countries, both developed and developing countries would be facing the future with much greater confidence and would be less worried about the economic implications of more elderly people.

The manifestations of the world recession which are most visible in the developed countries are rapid inflation and a high level of unemployment. Jobs are not being found for a high and socially damaging proportion of young people reaching working age. In the developed countries the percentage of the labor force without a job varies somewhat, but is around 10% – and official figures generally underestimate the real demand for jobs, particularly among women. What these countries are finding intolerable is to pay the cost of unemployment on top of the cost of the old and the young. Moreover, whereas in the 1950s many countries were cutting defence expenditure as they increased social spending, some countries are now loading extra defence expenditures on top of their increased social spending.

The public cost of unemployment and of devices to keep down the numbers on the published toll of unemployed is never fully totalled. First, there is the cost of supporting the unemployed on benefit or social assistance. Second, there is the loss of revenue to tax and social security funds. Third, there is the cost of special schemes of training and work experience. Fourth, there is the cost of subsidies to keep jobs going – including deficits in public enterprises such as public transport, airlines, and steel mills. Fifth, there is a whole variety of export subsidies. Sixth, there are the payments to workers made redundant.

The high rates of unemployment have been accompanied by inflation, which has eroded the value both of the private savings of the elderly and of their income from private pension schemes. As a result, many of the elderly who expected a standard of living not far below that which they had enjoyed in working life are faced with relative hardship. The effects fall most heavily on the very old, who are also the hardest hit by the higher relative cost of fuel, since they spend a greater proportion of their income on heating.

The world economic crisis has also had drastic consequences for the developing countries. Not only has the rise in oil prices reduced their capacity to import goods and skills needed for their development, but foreign aid has been drastically cut. The weak world market for raw materials has increased unemployment and underemployment, and has also eroded a critical part of their tax base. Some have been unable to import enough food to prevent famine. In addition, slow growth, no growth, or negative growth, coupled with ever-increasing public expenditure, have often cut into personal living standards. Many developing countries have been forced to devalue their currencies, thus raising the home price of imported goods and further reducing living standards.

As the experts who took part in this survey have sensed, this is not the economic climate in which governments are likely to launch costly new programs to promote the welfare of the elderly. Indeed, the trend is in the reverse direction. Where pensions have been indexed, some plans have been modified to give pensioners less than they had been led to expect. In countries where pensions have been locked into rigid financing systems, it can readily be foreseen that future commitments cannot be met if a substantial proportion of those of working age continue to have no work income from which to pay contributions, and if the level of work income stops increasing or starts to fall.

The trend to lower pension ages, in the hope of creating more jobs for younger people and hiding the real extent of underemployment, makes the problem of financing pensions still worse. The pensions of the early retired may finally be found by giving less to older pensioners. Though the extent to which early retirement does release jobs for younger people varies between different countries, it is clear that less than a full new job is created for each older worker who leaves the labor market. Another way of financing more pensions is to increase social charges, but this might deter potential investors from creating new jobs.

Will the crisis persist?

Thus the critical problem for the future of the elderly, as for others, is the state of the world economy. Is there a serious prospect that the present economic recession will persist for another 20 years? To me, such an assumption seems very unlikely for two reasons. First, no interpretation of past economic trends suggests a 20-year downturn in the trade cycle. Second, and more important, the present world imbalance of trade poses problems for everyone. It is because everyone stands to gain that I am confident that a solution will eventually be found. While growth in the next two decades may not be as rapid as it was in the past two decades, my guess is that by 1990 unemployment in the developed countries will be down to a tolerable level.

Retirement age

If one takes, as I do, an optimistic view of the longer-term future of the world economy, what consequences does this have for policy for the elderly? First, it seems to me highly undesirable to take decisions now to reduce retirement age which it would be extremely hard to reverse later on. Retirement age should be regarded as a social issue rather than an economic one. Moreover, longer-term economic considerations point in the same direction as social considerations. What is needed above all else is choice of age of retirement. People age at different rates. Some have poor health and others good health in their sixties. Moreover, some people have physically demanding and unpleasant jobs which they cannot, or do not want to, continue into old age. Others enjoy, if not always their jobs, at least the companionship and status which go with them. Many look forward to retiring, until the time when they are actually faced with this experience.

In the agricultural communities of developing countries, the elderly are able to work flexibly at those tasks which they are still able to do. Their knowledge gained from long experience is respected. The challenge for the developed countries is to secure a similar flexibility of work opportunity for their elders. For most people this is better than creating artificial roles and occupations. And as developing countries industrialize they need to find ways of building in their traditional flexibility on retirement practices. It is often forgotten that retirement at a specific age is largely a development of the twentieth century. The mistake so many developed countries have made is to build rigid retirement ages into pension schemes, in order to simplify personnel practices rather than to meet the wishes of individual employees, for whom the schemes were designed. The older worker should have legal rights to continue to work, not necessarily at the same job, long past the average age of retirement – and possibly also to "de-retire" and return to his old employer. Similarly, those who wish to retire earlier than the average, for health or other reasons, should have a real opportunity to do so in terms of pension rights. There should be arrangements for older workers to make a transition to retirement by part work and part pension.

Jobs caring for the elderly

Some argue that, even if economic growth resumes, there will not be jobs for everyone as we move into the age of micro-electronics. If job opportunities are short, then a shorter working week, paternity leave, sabbatical leave, and longer holidays are infinitely better social options than compulsorily depriving older people who want to continue to work at their jobs. And it is in the care of the old and disabled, and in preventing their exclusion from the rest of society, that there is such great potential for job creation – if ways can be found to fund the jobs. And this again depends on economic growth, as we learnt from the experience of the prosperous 1950s and 1960s. Moreover, the elderly themselves can make a major contribution to the lives of their families if they live near or with them.

Avoiding segregation

The second social lesson which is being re-learnt in the developed countries is that the elderly do not want to be excluded from the rest of society in institutions or retirement ghettos, however luxurious. The aim must be to enable them to remain in their own homes as long as possible, and thereafter in their own local environment, near family and friends. The aim of policy should be to make this possible by supporting and not supplanting the family. This is, moreover, not only socially desirable, as the international experts have pointed out – it is economically desirable as well. This policy will usually be cheaper than institutional care.

In many developed countries it is no longer acceptable to expect younger people, particularly women, to abandon their work careers because they have aged parents to care for. The main burden of caring will have to fall on paid staff, but families should not be made to feel that they cannot also help because they lack professional qualifications or training. In developing countries families do more. Moreover, there are less opportunities for paid work. The separation of families, due to job opportunities and the type of housing provided near places of work, must be avoided as far as possible. Some forms of social housing, as well as some forms of housing provided by employers, have the effect of breaking up families and dispersing communities, and thus destroying supportive social networks. This often happens when slums are cleared or shanty towns destroyed. The elderly must be able to live near or with their families. This principle has major implications for the siting of new economic activities. The aim must be to limit the growth of cities, and to avoid concentrating industry in one part of the country. Economic development must not be allowed to impose disproportionate social and economic burdens on society, and to generate needs for new services to replace the social support which has been destroyed.

Cost-effective health care

While the cost of providing pensions and social care for the elderly will not be beyond the capacity of developed economies with modest rates of growth, if the scourge of growing unemployment can be eliminated, there are some who argue that the cost of providing health care for the entire population, including the elderly, is bound to stretch economic resources beyond tolerable limits. They point out that technological progress in medicine has been one of the powerful forces making health-care costs rise faster than the rate of economic growth; this is bound to continue and, as noted earlier, the elderly are the largest users of health care. Against such reasoning are the following considerations.

First, it is not widely appreciated how small a role the increasing proportion of elderly in the population has been playing in increasing health-care costs. The changing demographic structure of the population has only added about 1% per annum, or less, of real growth to health-care costs over the past 30 years in developed countries which have long provided comprehensive and free, or virtually free, health care to the elderly. This explains only a small part of the doubling to quadrupling of real health-care expenditure in developed countries over the past 30 years.

Second, many technological developments in medicine have been introduced without careful evaluation of their effectiveness. Third, many countries have allowed expensive equipment to be provided so extensively that it is grossly under-used. Fourth, many procedures, such as pathological tests and drug therapy, are wastefully prescribed; moreover, in some countries iatrogenic disease is becoming a serious problem.

The accumulating evidence of the extent of unnecessary and inefficient use of health-care resources over the past 20 years is already leading to measures to control costs and improve efficiency. These measures are bound to become more effective over the next 20 years. More and more countries are regulating the number of hospital beds and the purchase of expensive equipment. There is a trend to establish a systematic evaluation of new technological developments before they are widely applied, and to look again at the appropriateness of older technologies. More and more countries are refusing to allow health-care costs to continue to increase at rates established in the past.

The World Health Organization is promoting primary health care as a means of providing more appropriate and cheaper health care in both developed and developing countries. The main thrust of health policy in the future must be directed towards disease prevention and health promotion. Many needs for health care can be avoided or postponed by changes in lifestyle and improvements in the economic and social environment. Developing countries can avoid the mistakes which the more developed countries have made, and establish health policies which are both more effective and more appropriate not only for the elderly but for other age groups.

A question which is of particular importance, in terms of both costs and ethics, concerns death. How far is it right to use modern health technology to strive to keep alive elderly people who no longer have any prospect of even a minimal quality of life? Should we allow the aged and seriously infirm to die in dignity, as is still the practice for most of the aged in developing countries? How should such decisions be made? These questions are bound to be pressed more strongly over the next 20 years. Practice already differs considerably according to the customs and ethics of the medical profession, the attitudes of relatives, and the legal provisions in different societies.

Pensions in developing countries

While developing countries can build up services for the elderly on a pattern which is both more socially desirable and more cost-effective than those which have generally evolved in developed countries, the most difficult problem is pensions. At what stage in development should pension schemes be initiated? For whom should they provide? Should they be funded or "pay-as-you-go"? How should they be financed? What should be the role of social assistance? In so far as pensions are funded, they accumulate savings to help push forward the process of development. On the other hand, the contributions that make up the fund can damage exports by raising labor costs.

It is generally agreed that reducing the rate of population growth is one of the most important means of raising living standards in the longer run. But to reduce population growth it is not enough to make family planning services readily available and to launch publicity campaigns to encourage their use. In some societies people want large families for good, logical reasons. One of them is to insure against isolation and destitution in old age. If families became smaller, none of the children may survive to care for their parents. Thus measures to increase the survival rates of children, and measures to guarantee the aged a minimum of security – if only by social assistance – can help to secure the acceptance of family planning services.

In developed countries, declines in birth rate have been accompanied by the growth of security in old age. And as families have become smaller, more provision for old age has become public rather than private. The precise relationship between pensions and family size cannot be proved beyond doubt, or predicted for all societies. There is no certainty that improved social provision for the elderly, taken by itself, will reduce the birth rate, and any such effects may be spread over a long period. On the other hand, it is wrong to go to the other extreme and regard provision for the elderly as in all cases a wasteful diversion of funds which could be used for promoting development and improving the prospects of the young. Security in old age may, in some societies, help to secure the acceptance of family planning, lower birth rates, and higher living standards in the future.

Conclusion

But it remains true that improved provisions for the elderly are unlikely to be made while the present world economic crisis persists. The heavy costs of the crisis, for both developed and developing countries, limit the acceptability of increases in public expenditure. But if the crisis can be overcome and modest economic growth resumed, the balance between working population and dependants, including the higher proportion of the elderly, will not impose insuperable "burdens" on the economies of the more developed countries. Developing countries will still, inevitably, be faced with difficult problems in establishing their priorities for public expenditure. They can, however, at least learn from the experience of the more developed countries what to avoid. The aim of policy must be to hold the family together as far as possible, to develop community rather than institutional services, and to avoid inappropriate or unnecessarily expensive services. Moreover, greater security for the elderly may contribute to socio-economic development and thereby benefit later generations.

Brian Abel-Smith,
professor of social administration,
London School of Economics
and Political Science

A statement from WHO

Three general principles and ten specific principles are proposed, as a framework for formulating policies and programs on aging within overall national plans.

General principles

To establish health and social policies on aging, the key issues must be brought into the political arena. The following general principles are directed at political decision makers.

1. Policies for people

Health and development policies express the political will of governments to do something for people, with people. Aging policies reflect the commitment of governments to maintain the elderly within society in a state that gives dignity both to elderly individuals and to the community.

2. Triumph of survival

It would be a perversity to consider the results of our increasing success in improving human survival, and in regulating fertility, as problems. Rather, wise and far-sighted statesmen should try to foresee what these twin triumphs of 20th century civilization imply for life on our planet, now and in the year 2000. We are entering an age of aging. The effect of this on societies should be viewed positively, as a triumph and not as a problem.

3. Advancing our humanity

A principle underlying all social policies should be that the whole of mankind is devalued when any group of human beings is devalued on grounds of race, religion, sex, or age. A general consensus on this principle has been established among nations over the past three decades. The sustained international effort to advance humanity passes a further historic milepost with the United Nations World Assembly on Aging. This gathering may mark the beginning of the end of age discrimination in human society.

Specific principles

1. Sharing the benefits of societal development

All human rights and privileges should extend to the elderly. Many elderly people, by virtue of a lifetime characterized by war, struggle, and hardship, have a special claim to a fair share of the benefits flowing from the development of our societies. Beyond material needs, the elderly require at least as much social interaction, emotional support, and care as the rest of society.

The well-being of people in old age is determined by the conditions of life during their working years. Inequalities during this earlier phase of life are perpetuated and even aggravated with aging. Thus, policies for the elderly should not be formulated without reference to the needs of other age groups in the same society. In particular, resources must be allocated preferentially to the most economically deprived people, whatever their age. The coming generation of elderly people will benefit from continuing efforts to reduce health inequalities and to achieve "health for all by the year 2000".

2. Individuality of elderly persons

The population described as elderly is not a homogeneous group. Indeed, the variation in individual capacities increases with age. From the health perspective, those aged 60 and over comprise two generations – a younger and generally fit group, and an older group that is especially vulnerable to health impairments.

3. Independence

The keystone of policies on aging is the commitment of all sectors of government, of non-governmental organizations, of the caring professions, and of individuals to programs aimed at the promotion of health and the maintenance of function during aging. Impaired health, aggravated by social and economic disadvantages, diminishes the activity of elderly people, reduces their independence, incapacitates them, and affects the quality of their life.

Services should not generate dependence, and paternalistic practices which erode independence should be discarded. An explicit objective of health policies should be to help elderly persons maintain the maximum degree of independent life in the face of increasing difficulty in performing daily activities.

The principle of promoting and maintaining independence applies also to housing, transportation, and social and family-welfare policies.

4. Choice

All too often, the Third Age is the "age of no consent". Decisions affecting elderly citizens are frequently made without their participation. This applies particularly to those who are very old, frail, or disabled. Such people should be served by flexible systems of care that give them a choice of types of amenities and care. In particular, the elderly should not cede control of their own lives to health, social-service, and other caring personnel, since they themselves usually know best what is needed and how it should be carried out.

5. Home care

In 1978, WHO member states adopted a policy, expressed in the Declaration of Alma-Ata, of providing primary health care. This is defined as essential health care which is based on practical, scientifically sound, and socially acceptable methods, and which is universally accessible to individuals and families in the community through their full participation. From this policy there stems an unequivocal commitment to supporting and caring for persons of advanced age within their own homes.

Developing countries will be unable to afford the costs of institutional care. They should therefore establish policies of community-based care for the elderly. Home care is the best economic option, and also provides more emotional satisfaction.

Contrary to widespread belief, a considerable proportion of mental disorders in old age are either treatable, partly preventable, or modifiable by means that require neither specialized nor institutional care.

6. Accessibility

Public services should be accessible to all generations. In addition to health services, leisure, recreational, and educational facilities

189

need to be progressively adapted to cater for all generations, not only for younger people. The early development of leisure, recreational, and educational activities that help people to prepare for retirement is of particular importance.

7. Engaging the elderly

Policies should aim to promote cohesion between the generations. The application of this principle to the area of health means that elderly individuals, their families, and neighbors would share responsibility for adopting health measures aimed at improving the health and well-being of the community as a whole. Another consequence for health programs might be that the elderly would help young or disabled people, as in the "adopted grandparent" projects of some countries.

Housing policies aimed at re-uniting the generations would help to create better-balanced communities blending different age groups.

8. Mobility

The elderly, particularly in rural areas, are often unable to use public amenities and services because of impaired mobility. A first priority for informal good neighborliness, or for lay and religious volunteer activity, should be to assist elderly citizens to achieve sufficient mobility to enable them to attend local markets, shopping areas, community centers, religious services, and primary health care facilities.

Elderly people who need help to keep themselves mobile would benefit from the advice of caring personnel who are trained to assess functional capacity and to offer guidance on adaptations and aids to daily living.

9. Productivity

The great majority of elderly people today do not show symptoms of decline in their mental and physical function, but rather enjoy a level of health that permits them to lead a socially and economically productive life. In the developed world, an increasing number of people of all ages are committed to healthier eating habits and lifestyles, and to the maintenance of physical fitness, mental alertness, and a stimulating social environment. These future cohorts, of people who retain their health but retire from the work force, represent a vast resource of skilled and experienced people – one which no society can afford to leave untapped. More flexibility is required in the distribution of work over the life-span, while education needs to be viewed as a continuous, life-long process.

Public and private employers, trade unions, educational bodies, voluntary agencies, and elderly self-help groups should organize programs to provide the stimulus and motivation to develop a purposeful life after retirement.

10. Self-care and care by the family

Elderly people, together with their families, should be more involved in their own care. Information is required on the promotion of health and the prevention of disease, as are simple handbooks of personal care. Knowledge of locally available services and social support systems is also important, and will assist elderly people and their families in seeking health care. Too often the elderly fail to seek care, in the belief that ailments are part of the aging process.

Public authorities should identify and support people who are caring for frail, elderly relatives at home, since this often imposes heavy physical, emotional, and financial demands.

New orientations are required on the part of care providers – to help elderly people maintain independence, to promote self-care, and to prevent disability. Such support to the elderly requires practitioners who are knowledgeable about aging, who are interested in elderly people and their families, who are skilled in working with them, and who are concerned about the quality of care given.

Leo A. Kaprio,
regional director,
World Health Organization,
regional office for Europe,
Copenhagen

A view from the UN

There is something intriguing about the concepts of aging and old age as they are commonly perceived today. Our ambivalent attitude towards aging, as a social phenomenon and as a personal predicament, seems to be rooted in vague and contradictory ideas of what aging is, and of what it is to be aging. As a result, both personal attitudes and public policies need analysis and clarification.

This is particularly so in the more developed countries, which have undergone impressive changes in their demographic structure during the last decades. The aging of societies, in terms of both increasing individual longevity and the relative proportion of elderly people, implies that the prospect of surviving well beyond retirement age, which once was the privilege of the few, has now become almost a certainty for most people. For society, the number and proportion of old people – too many to be taken care of in the traditional family context – have become social and economic problems of the first order.

However, as implied by the comments of several experts quoted in this book, this process seems to have been accompanied by a growing discrepancy between two incompatible perceptions – of aging as a phenomenon, and of the elderly as a group. On the one hand, aging is "for all", as a present reality or a close prospect. As a predicament, it is quite different from, say, being male or female, black or white, rich or poor, handicapped or able-bodied – categories to which one belongs independently of choice, or into which one may happen to fall by chance. Growing older – except for the very few who choose to opt out before their time – is a part of every human life, and indeed of all biological existence. The aged are all of us, now or later, without any real or imagined ground for discrimination. But the sad paradox is that policies for the protection of the aged, created with the best of humanitarian motives, have in themselves become a ground for discrimination – against ourselves, as it were.

The author's comments are made in a personal capacity and do not necessarily reflect the position of the United Nations.

Modern industrial societies, with elaborate social-security systems, tend to *define* a person into old age by a certain pre-established point in life. Retirement from full-time gainful employment, even when financial security in the later years of life is guaranteed, has become the artificial cut-off point from what, too often, is seen as the main or only useful function a person can have in society. It is almost a reverse form of initiation rites into adulthood, practiced in many societies. Instead of growing older, the individual is forced into a category called "aged" or "elderly". This tends to be conceived of as a homogeneous group – a special, and somehow different, breed of human beings with shared and unique characteristics.

Most people, however, would subscribe to the remark made by one of the experts quoted in this book: "At no other stage in life are the differences between individuals more marked than in old age." This remark has a double intent. If "old age" is taken to be the period between retirement and death, it refers, at least in the more developed regions, to an average span of several decades – a period during which the differences between the "young old" and the "old old" may be as marked as those between an adolescent and a person of middle age. Furthermore, the natural accumulation of life experience, good or bad, produces a diversity of attitudes, interests, and self-perception which, for the individual, is infinitely more important than the consciousness of being one among the "old".

This, of course, goes for personal expectations as well. Those of us who are still some years away from retirement rarely think of our own aging, if we give it any thought at all, in terms of joining a faceless mass called the elderly, or of letting ourselves be co-opted into another category of human beings. Whatever changes in living conditions and re-adjustments may be foreseen, it will not be *we* who change, except maybe in the very long run. Our own way of life, interests, and idiosyncrasies will continue to define us, with the label "aged" as an imposed and marginal addition. And we naturally expect others – relatives, friends, and the community around us – to perceive and relate to us in the same manner.

We are therefore faced with a discrepancy of ideas and perceptions about aging which, far more than practical issues of policies and actions, request our attention at this stage. As long as everybody, from governments and policy-makers to individual experts and the public at large, maintains a double standard towards aging and the elderly, based on incompatible views such as those outlined above, no rational policy at national or international level can be formulated. The creation of broad, formalized social-security systems has been a first and important step in providing for the elderly. It was based on

– and at the same time created – the concept of aging as a final step in life, and of the retired elderly as a category apart. The inherent shortcomings of these systems, and of the way of social thinking which they unwittingly entail, are in stark contrast to individual realities and social objectives.

Social policies that do not reflect and respond to existing realities – as perceived individually and collectively – are bound to fail, in one way or another. Failure does not necessarily mean that stated goals are not attained. It may also mean over-attainment or, more typically, unwanted and unforeseen side effects. This seems to have been the case with generalized policies for the protection of the aged. Their justified quest for equal rights and coverage was inevitably based on a rigid definition of aging in terms of compulsory retirement ages, with consequent rights and benefits for persons attaining a certain age and/or length of service.

It is striking to observe that, in the views of experts from a large number of countries quoted in this book, the magnitude of the problem of caring for the elderly is only one source of concern. The qualitative aspect plays an almost equal part. Needs to improve financial security, health, and mental alertness are seen as new problems in a society which no longer imposes upon the retired person material dependency and social marginalization. This is yet another recognition of the deep contrast between policies based on a generalized idea of the aged as a homogeneous group, and the more intuitive and realistic understanding that this is nothing but a fiction – that the conditions, needs, and capacities of the aged are as diverse as those of any other part of the population.

Our main problem perhaps is that the aging of our societies has come about too early, and out of step with goals of material, technological, social, and psychological progress during the last few centuries. Advances in medicine, both preventive and curative, figure as the main villain here – they have too far outpaced progress in material living conditions, the distribution of resources and opportunities, and social justice in general. In the less developed countries, people will in future live longer but equally miserable lives. People in more developed countries can expect even longer, healthier, and more fulfilling lives, tempered by other forms of misery in their later years.

Is this progress? It certainly is, if we consider that a long life – and preferably a happy and comfortable long life – has forever been a mainstay of human imagination and striving, inspiring whatever efforts have been made to improve our lot. The aging of societies, despite all the accompanying imbalances and set-backs, is one of mankind's most concrete and visible triumphs in its efforts to secure a better life for every individual. Once its contradictions and problems are worked out, it should rank higher as a human achievement than any other form of technological or material progress.

"If there is a basis for pessimism about the future, there also is a basis for optimism: the forces that produce longer life and vigor can be harnessed to reduce or eliminate the problems that have accompanied them." In these words, the overall summary of this book (see p. 17) puts the argument in a nutshell. Aging, both as individual fate and as social concern, is more than a "problem" – it is a positive challenge, and should be taken as such by the individual and by society. We have all wanted it, and have to make the best of it.

Two rather distressing facts should be taken into account here. As observed above, the introduction of social-security arrangements based on fixed and compulsory retirement ages entailed an artificial split between the active and passive sectors of the population. This was dictated by practical and administrative necessities, and inspired by concerns for equality and social justice. It did not, in itself, define the onset of old age – it merely attributed certain rights to individuals having reached a certain stage in life, or a certain number of years of employment. The juxtaposition of retirement with entry into old age is something imposed by public thinking – by the reactions of beneficiaries of retirement schemes, as well as by their relatives and communities. The process of being "defined" into old age at the point of retirement is a result not only of administrative action but also of public attitudes, which have somehow sanctioned this artificial device as a "real" transition into a state of dependency and social marginality. By this perverse acceptance of the officially defined point of entry into old age, we have done a great disservice to the elderly of today and tomorrow – that is, to ourselves.

The second distressing fact is that we tend to shrink from any personal responsibility for this state of affairs, and to expect the State, or the community at large, if not friends or relatives, to make up for the adverse effects of retirement and entry into so-called old age. Strictly speaking, the State and the community have fulfilled their responsibility towards the aging individual by providing for his or her financial security, health care, and other basic needs. Happiness and contentment cannot be provided by any outside agency or public program – at best, these can help to shield the individual from poverty and other direct sources of unhappiness. Like everyone else, the aging individual must assume responsibility for his or her own life.

A main purpose of the World Assembly on Aging is to draw attention to the rapid aging of the world's population. Most of us will outlive our so-called productive years, and will then have to face up to years or decades of post-retirement existence. In this context, the idea of "preparing for retirement" is a much more serious proposition than just another subject for evening classes or manuals advising those about to retire. Preparation for retirement, which may well cover up to a third of the life-span, should become a life-long concern of individuals and societies — a part of education, training, and other forms of preparation for life.

For the great mass of individuals, especially in the more developed countries, this would require nothing short of a revolution in prevailing attitudes, ideas, and expectations about life itself. So long as the value of a person continues to be measured in terms of employment status, social roles, and income, the misery of being pushed aside at a certain age is no more than just retribution for a distorted and short-sighted view of what human life is all about. Family and friends, social relationships, hobbies and personal interests — everything which could, and should, occupy a person's life as much as a salaried job or a formal social status — are not lost at the age of retirement. Rather, their value and importance are enhanced. The most important things in life can be achieved by a person who is free to give them full and exclusive attention.

At some point in the future a balance must, and will, be found. The sheer numbers of the elderly, if not a radical change of attitudes and values, will create awareness of the fact that modern societies are largely composed of people who have fulfilled their roles in the productive system but can continue to maintain all other social roles, duties, and responsibilities. This would be a great achievement in the world-wide effort to create a better life for all. We are well on the way to ensuring that everybody has a chance to survive into old age. The challenge now is to make that into a worth-while prospect.

Eyvind Hytten,
special advisor to the
secretary-general of the
World Assembly on Aging,
United Nations,
Vienna

STATISTICS

List of Tables and Figures

Population in millions (total, aged 60+, 70+, 80+) (1980–2000)

	Total population			Population 60+			Population 70+			Population 80+		
	1980	2000	Increase %	1980	2000	Increase %	1980	2000	Increase %	1980	2000	Increase %
Australia	14·5	17·8	23	1·9	2·7	38·7	0·8	1·3	58·7	0·2	0·3	61·4
Brazil	122·3	187·5	53	7·5	14·0	86·7	3·0	6·0	100·0	0·7	1·6	117·1
Egypt	42·0	64·4	53	2·4	4·6	91·7	0·8	1·7	112·5	0·1	0·3	146·9
Federal Republic of Germany	60·9	58·8	−3	11·4	13·3	16·9	6·0	6·1	1·1	1·5	1·7	12·8
France	53·5	56·3	5	9·1	10·8	19·4	5·1	5·6	10·4	1·4	1·5	4·9
India	684·5	960·6	40	33·9	65·7	93·8	11·1	22·4	101·8	2·0	3·6	80·0
Israel	3·9	5·6	44	0·4	0·6	38·2	0·2	0·3	50·0	0·04	0·08	100·0
Italy	56·9	59·1	4	10·0	13·5	34·6	5·0	6·9	38·0	1·2	1·9	55·5
Japan	116·6	129·3	11	14·8	26·4	78·4	6·4	11·9	85·9	1·5	3·0	102·5
Kenya	16·5	30·4	84	0·7	1·3	85·7	0·3	0·5	66·7	0·04	0·1	150·0
Nigeria	77·1	150·0	95	3·1	6·4	106·5	1·0	2·2	120·0	0·2	0·4	155·3
Philippines	49·2	77·0	57	2·2	4·6	109·1	0·7	1·7	142·9	0·1	0·3	114·5
Poland	35·8	41·2	15	4·7	6·8	44·7	2·3	3·2	39·1	0·5	0·7	50·0
Sweden	8·3	8·1	−2	1·8	1·8	−1·8	0·9	1·0	11·1	0·2	0·3	36·9
United Kingdom	55·9	55·2	−1	11·1	11·3	1·3	5·4	6·0	11·1	1·4	1·8	28·6
USA	223·2	263·8	18	33·9	40·1	18·3	15·6	20·6	32·1	4·4	5·8	31·8
World	4,432·1	6,118·8	38	375·8	590·4	57·1	158·3	252·3	59·5	35·3	59·6	68·8

Source: Provisional projections of the United Nations Population Division, New York, 1980.

199

FIGURE 1

Percentage of population aged 60+ (1980–2000)

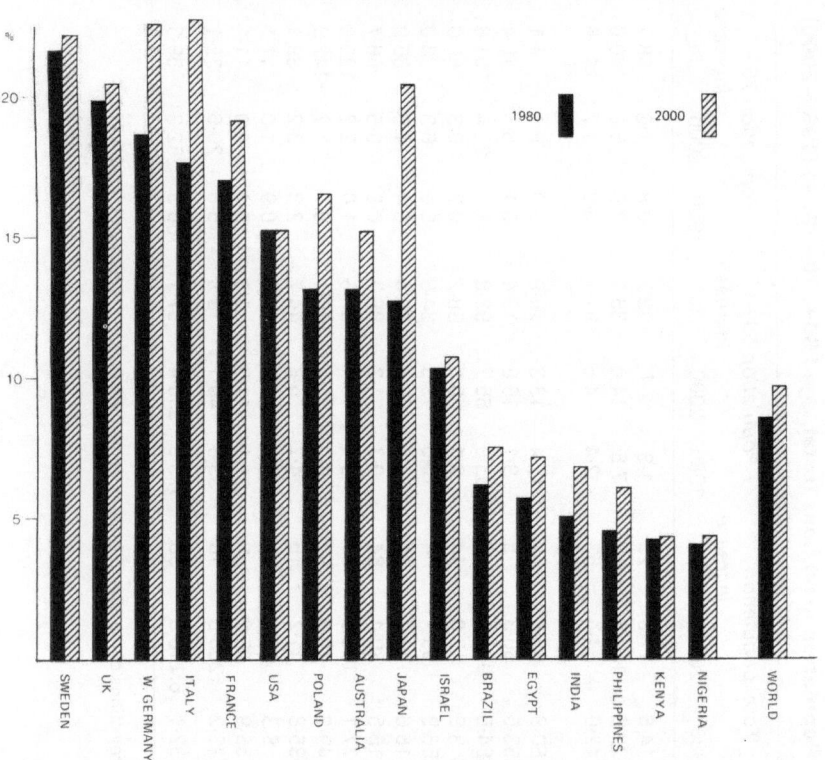

Source: Provisional projections of the United Nations Population Division, New York, 1980.

FIGURE 2

Percentage of population aged 80+ (1980–2000)

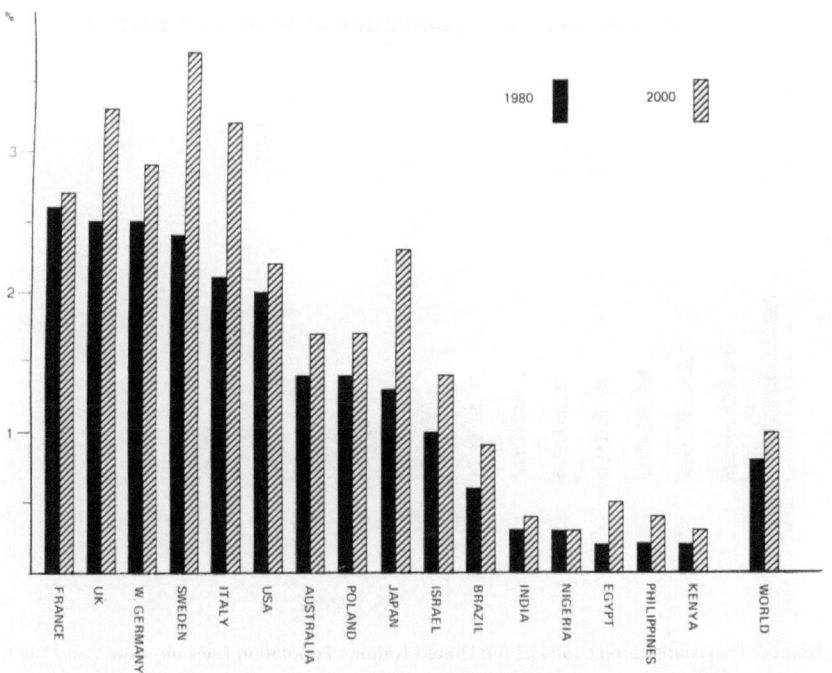

Source: Provisional projections of the United Nations Population Division, New York, 1980.

FIGURE 3

Percentage of women in population aged 60+ (1980–2000)

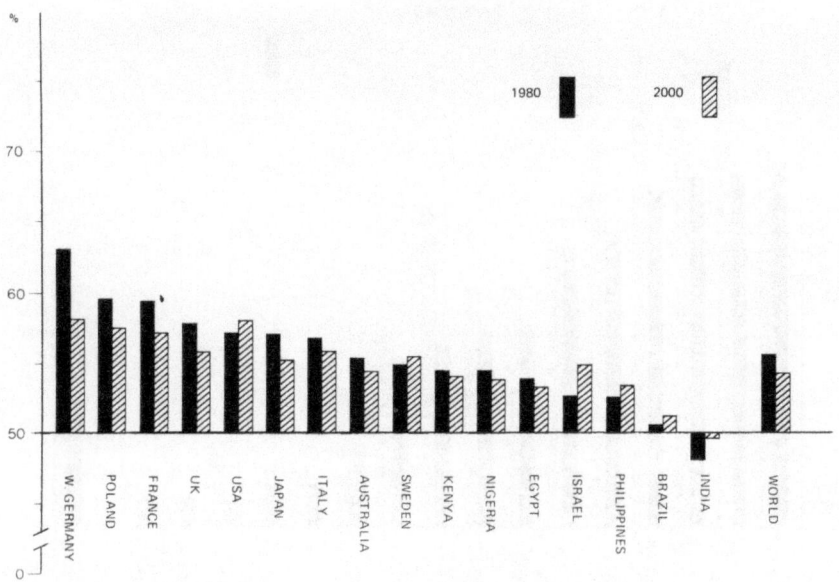

Source: Provisional projections of the United Nations Population Division, New York, 1980.

FIGURE 4

Percentage of women in population aged 80+ (1980–2000)

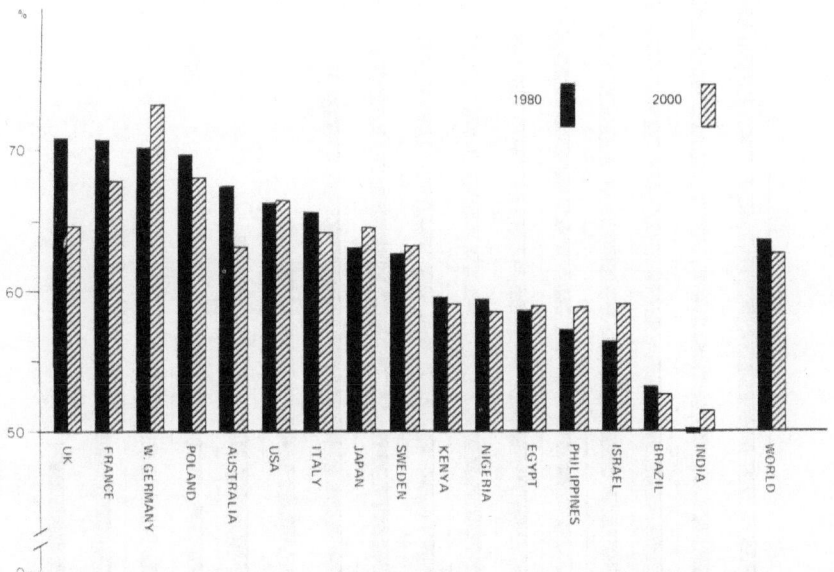

Source: Provisional projections of the United Nations Population Division, New York, 1980.

FIGURE 5

Life expectancy at birth (1975–80) for females and males

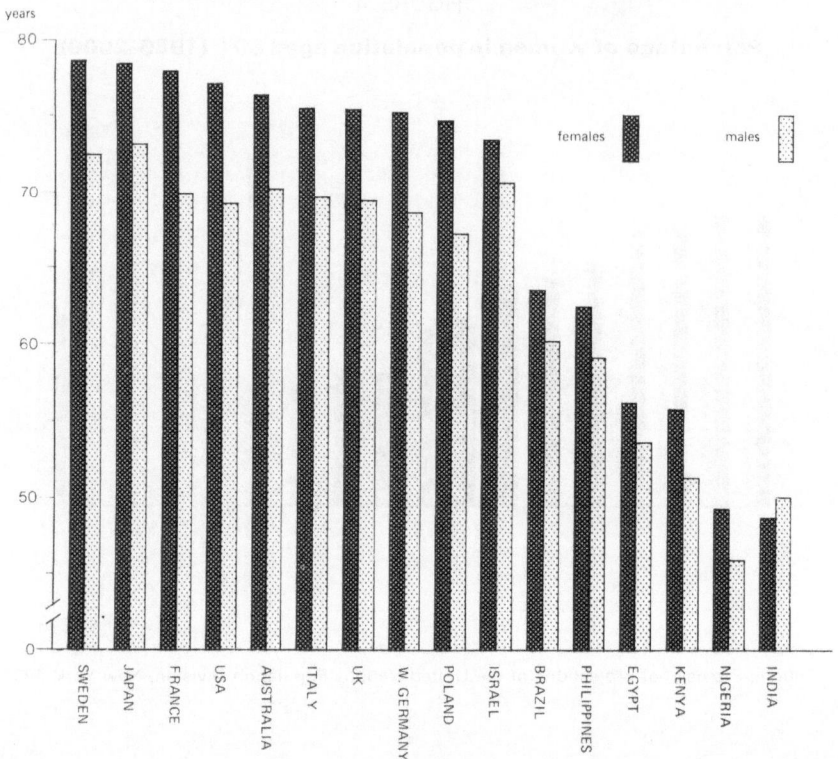

Source. Provisional projections of the United Nations Population Division, New York, 1980.

FIGURE 6

Life expectancy at age 60 (1975–80) for females and males

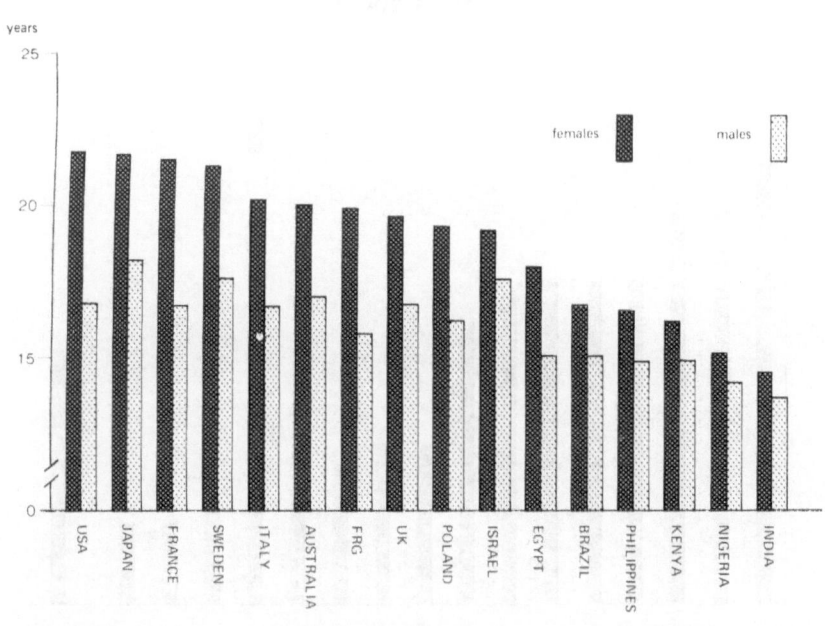

Sources:
(1) Calculated from Coale-Demeny West model life tables with life expectancies at birth from same source as Figure 5 (above) (for Australia, Brazil, India, Philippines, Poland, UK).
(2) United Nations, *Demographic Yearbook 1978* (Sales no. E/F.79.XIII.1), table 22 (for Egypt, Federal Republic of Germany, France, Israel, Italy, Sweden, USA).
(3) Japan, Bureau of Statistics, *Japan Statistical Yearbook 1980*, Tokyo, p. 41 (for Japan).
(4) Calculated using the Coale-Demeny North model life tables (for Kenya, Nigeria).

Note: Life expectancy is given for the period 1975–80, except for the following countries: Egypt (1960), Federal Republic of Germany (1975–77), France (1976), Israel (1977), Italy (1970–72), Japan (1978), Sweden (1972-76), USA (1975)

FIGURE 7

Percentage of men aged 65+ who are economically active (1980–2000)

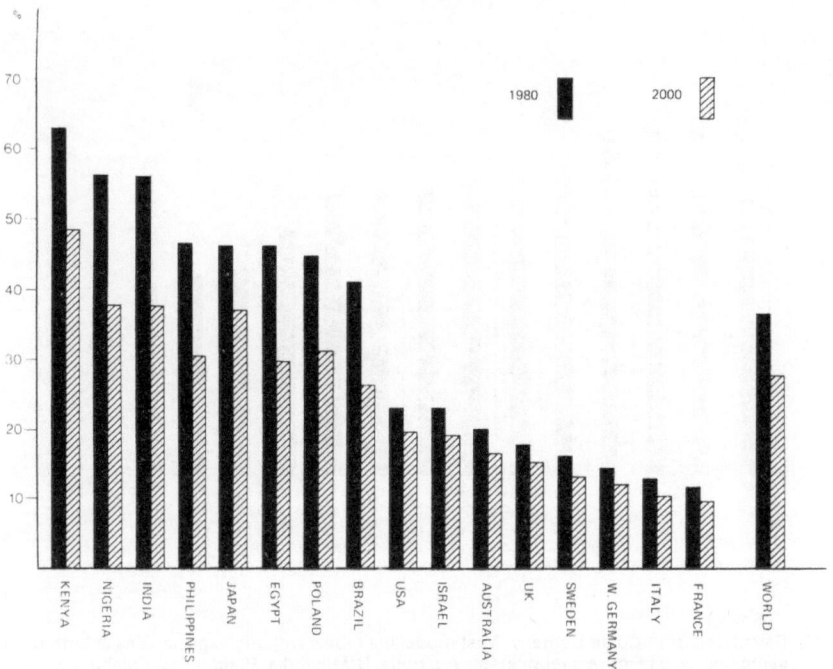

Source: International Labour Office (1977) 1950–2000 labour force: Estimates for the period 1950–1970, Projections for the period 1975–2000, Vol. I-V.

FIGURE 8

Percentage of women aged 65+ who are economically active (1980–2000)

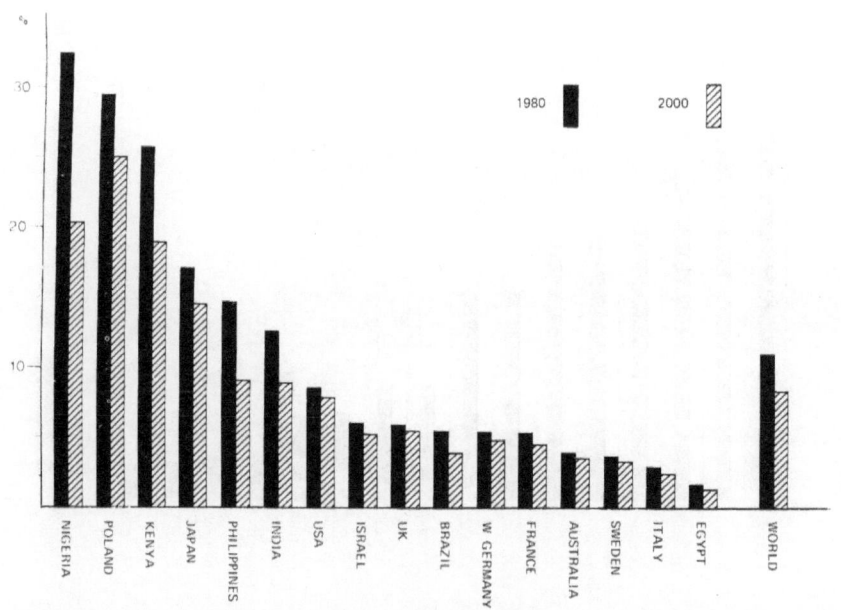

Source: International Labour Office (1977) 1950–2000 labour force: Estimates for the period 1950–1970, Projections for the period 1975–2000, Vol. I-V.

FIGURE 9

Economically non-active men aged 65+ as percentage of total economically active population (1980–2000)

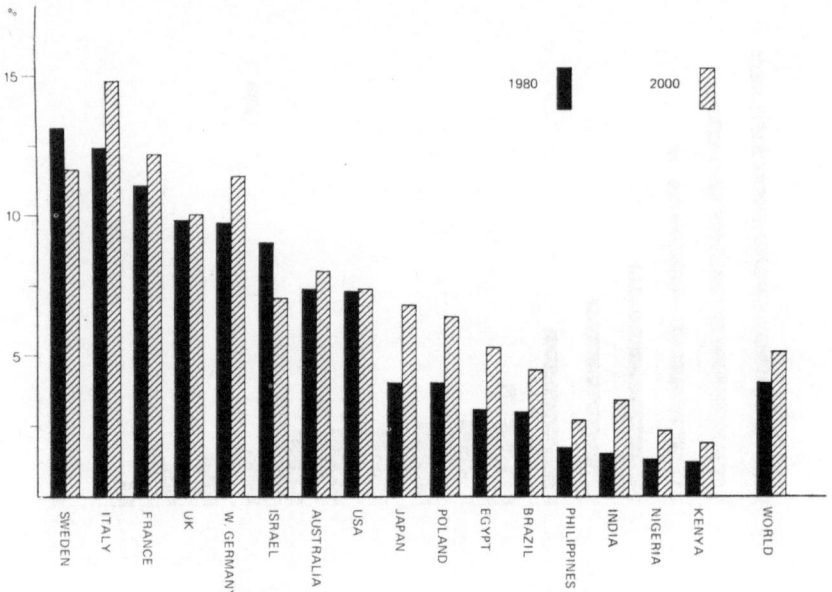

Source: International Labour Office (1977) 1950–2000 labour force: Estimates for the period 1950–1970, Projections for the period 1975–2000, Vol. I-V.

FIGURE 10

Economically non-active women aged 65+ as percentage of total economically active population (1980–2000)

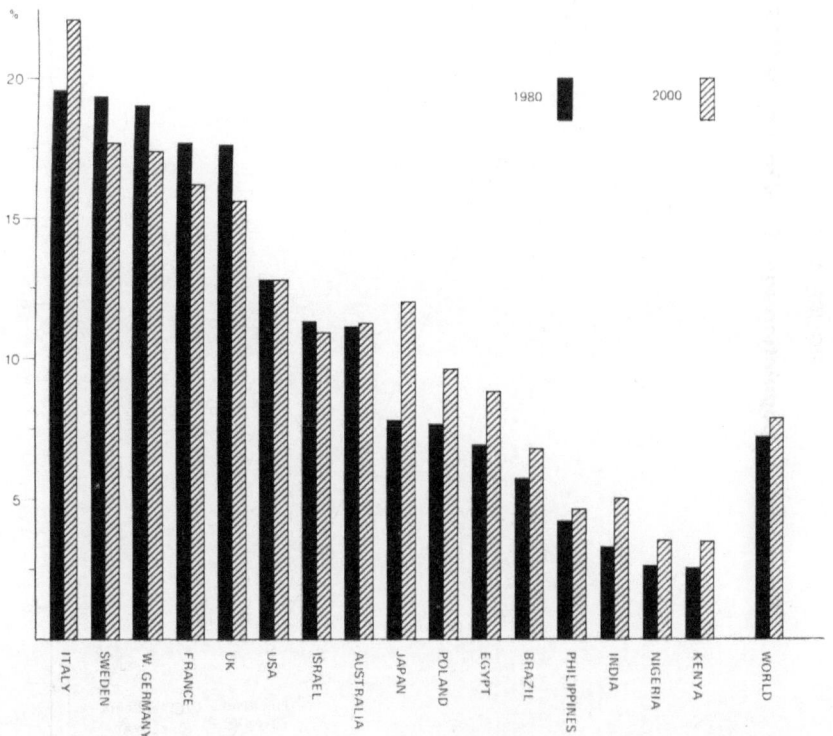

Source: International Labour Office (1977) 1950–2000 labour force: Estimates for the period 1950–1970, Projections for the period 1975–2000, Vol. I-V.

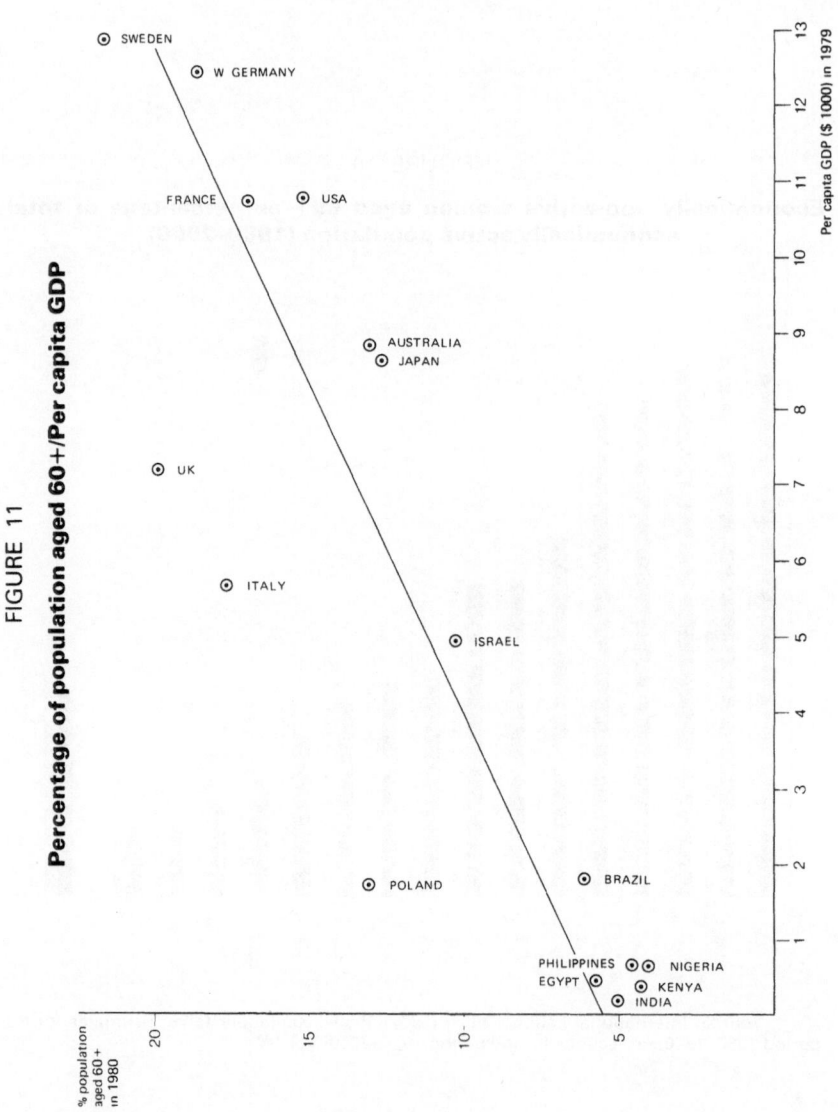

FIGURE 11

Percentage of population aged 60+/Per capita GDP

Sources.
(1) Same source as Figures 1–5 (above) (Percentage of population aged 60+).
(2) Figures supplied by the United Nations Statistical Office (Per capita GDP).

Note: For Nigeria, the per capita GDP in 1978 is given. For Poland, the per capita net material product is given.

Glossary

The following definitions are proposed in order to help the lay reader, and represent the usage of terms in this book. A comprehensive international glossary of terms in social gerontology is currently being prepared by the International Federation on Ageing.

Adult education – Organized learning to meet the needs of persons beyond compulsory school age.

Age cohort – Persons born during the same specified period of time.

Ageism – Prejudice against people because they are old.

Aging – The biological and psycho-social changes that occur normally as an individual becomes older.

Chronic disease, disability – A sickness (diabetes, arthritis) or limitation of function (low vision) that lasts a long time, The condition may require adjustment of an individual's life-style and the provision of medical, nursing, and social services.

Community-based services – Private or public health and social-support services given in the home, the provider's office, an outpatient clinic, or a communal meeting place. The term contrasts with services provided for patients as residents of a hospital or nursing home.

Community care – Any form of care of persons outside of an institution by means of health and social services based in the community.

Congregate housing – Apartment houses or other group accommodations in which health care and supporting services are provided as needed for the elderly who are functionally impaired but not routinely in need of nursing care, or who are socially deprived.

Continuum of care – The range of health and social-support services

211

required by individuals with progressive dependency due to loss of physical or mental capacity. Ideally, the services are provided without interruption as the patient's needs change.

Cross-sectional research – Research which compares individuals with different characteristics or conditions (eg, different ages) at one point in time. (See also longitudinal research.)

Day care – Social, recreational, and rehabilitative services provided in a supervised setting to persons who do not require institutional care but, because of physical or mental impairment, require day-time supervision. It may be provided in an adult day-care center, hospital, senior center, nursing home, or other community facility. Services may include treatment or activities to help improve physical and mental health. Meals and transportation may be provided.

Day hospital – A part of a hospital in which patients receive medical care and rehabilitation during the day and return home at night. Such facilities which treat older patients are often referred to as geriatric day hospitals.

Dementia – Impairment of thinking and memory.

Dependency ratio – The number of young and old individuals (below and above conventional working age) as a proportion of the population of conventional working age (18 – 64 years). The ratio gives a rough idea of the dependency "burden" that workers support. The elderly dependency ratio is the number of old individuals as a proportion of the population of conventional working age.

Elder, elderly – People who have reached the age of 60 or 65 years. The age of 60 years has been adopted by the United Nations for the purpose of the World Assembly on Aging.

Epidemiology – The study of the relationships of various physical, social, economic, and other factors determining the frequency and distribution of diseases in a population.

Flexible retirement – An option allowing an individual to retire at an age of his or her choice.

Functional age – An indicator of age based on physical or mental performance criteria, rather than on chronological age.

Functional capacity – The ability of an individual to accomplish a task despite physical or mental limitations. Sometimes the goal of treatment is to improve functional capacity of an individual whose disease or disability cannot be improved.

Geriatrics – A branch of medicine which is concerned with all aspects of health and health care of the elderly.

Geriatric assessment – A set of procedures for assessing an elderly person's physical and mental characteristics and determining services needed to improve ability to carry out the normal activities of living. It is used as a basis for a plan of care, and for monitoring the effects of prescribed services and activities in achieving treatment goals.

Gerontology – A multidisciplinary science concerned with processes of aging and the circumstances of the elderly in society.

Gradual retirement – Gradual reduction of the work time to ease the transition to full retirement (synonym: phased retirement).

Granny flat – A permanent or temporary accommodation adjoining a family home which enables an older person or persons to maintain independent living while remaining part of the family unit.

Health services – Services provided by professionals and others for prevention, diagnosis, treatment, and rehabilitation, and for health promotion and maintenance.

Home care – The provision of health and/or supportive services to enable an ill or disabled person to continue living at home.

Home for the aged – An institution for elderly people who need social support but who do not need regular nursing care.

Home health care – The provision of health services in the home, including nursing, physical, speech, and occupational therapy, and nutritional support.

Home help – A non-professional who is paid to help the individual or family with personal care and routine household tasks.

Hospice – A facility which cares for the dying person. It is designed to maximize the quality of life of dying patients and their families.

Institutionalization – Admission of an individual to an institution, such as a hospital or nursing home, for care requiring residence and for services usually unavailable in the outside community.

Inter-generational conflict – Conflict based on competition between old and young adults for limited social and economic resources.

Life cycle – The entire life course viewed as a progression from infancy to old age. Social roles and expectations, health, and socio-economic status tend to change typically as an individual moves from one phase to the next.

Life expectancy – The average number of years of life remaining to persons of a given age if current age-specific mortality rates continue. Life expectancy for people of the same age may vary according to socio-economic and other factors.

Longitudinal research – Study of the characteristics or conditions of the same individuals over a period of time. (See also cross-sectional research.)

Long-term care – The range of medical and social care for individuals having chronic functional impairment in activities of daily living. It may be provided by formal or informal support systems.

Mandatory retirement – The policy of requiring persons to leave employment with a particular firm or institution upon reaching a stated age.

Meals on wheels – The provision of home-delivered meals, often by a voluntary or philanthropic organization.

Nursing home – A long-term care facility that provides residential accommodation, nursing care, and other services for ill or disabled persons.

Phased retirement – Gradual reduction of the work time to ease the transition to full retirement (synonym: gradual retirement).

Preventive medicine – Activities designed to minimize the occurrence and progression of disease and disability, and to promote the well-being of individuals and the community. They include vaccination, nutrition counseling, screening, health education, and assessment of living habits.

Psycho-social research – Study of attitudes, social interactions, intellectual abilities, family relationships, and other factors that, as considered in this book, influence how people age.

Respite care – Short-term care under professional supervision, either at home or in an institution, to provide respite for the habitual care-giver.

Retirement – The act of leaving paid, full-time employment for the rest of one's life. However, a retiree may work irregularly or part-time. After retirement, a pension, or social-security or other regular payment, may be provided by the government or a private organization.

Self-help groups – Voluntary, small groups which provide mutual aid and support to members in dealing with their problems and concerns.

Senile dementia – A condition of unknown cause, characterized by brain atrophy and a progressive loss of mental function.

Senior center – A community facility which provides recreational, educational, cultural, and social activities, and minor health care, for the elderly.

Sheltered housing – (UK) Grouped independent accommodations linked to a warden's residence by alarm. Services are not provided. (USA) Synonymous with congregate housing.

Social services – Services which help individuals with personal problems of housing, transportation, meals, loneliness, family conflict, recreation, etc. They may be provided by social workers, community workers, ministers, lay persons, and family members.

Social-support system – Any system of interpersonal transactions which provide aid to others in the form of emotional support, approval, or goods and services. A formal system includes professional care-givers; an informal system includes non-professionals such as family members, friends, and neighbors.

List of Experts

AUSTRALIA

Prof. Gary ANDREWS — community health and geriatric medicine, The Parramatta Hospital, Westmead, NSW (HEALTH)

Dr Edward CULLEN — director of geriatrics, northern region, Health Commission of New South Wales, Chatswood, NSW (SOCIOLOGY)

Dr Sidney SAX — head, social welfare policy secretariat, Federal Department of Social Welfare, Woden, ACT (SOCIAL POLICY)

Mr Cliff PICTON — chief executive, Australian Council on the Aging, Melbourne (ADVISOR)

BRAZIL

Prof. Irany Novah MORAES — chairman, board of directors, university hospital, University of São Paulo (HEALTH)

Prof. Nai Lemos GONCALVES — deputy director, school of law, University of São Paulo (SOCIOLOGY)

Prof. Fernando Proenca de GOUVEIA — assessor to the secretary of health, State of São Paulo (SOCIAL POLICY)

EGYPT

Prof. Essam FIKRY — chairman, department of internal medicine, and chief, geriatric research center, faculty of medicine, University of Alexandria (HEALTH)

Mrs Haifaa SHANAWANY — consultant, Population and Family Planning Board, Cairo (SOCIOLOGY)

Mr Amin Ibrahim ALY — under-secretary of state, Ministry of Social Affairs, Cairo (SOCIAL POLICY)

Mrs Mary Fadel GUIRGUIS — gerontologist, American University, Cairo (MODERATOR)

Dr Fouad HENEIN — geriatrician, Heliopolis (ADVISOR)

Dr Mark C. KENNEDY — associate professor, departments of sociology, anthropology, and psychology, American University of Cairo (ADVISOR)

Mr Ahmed SHOUKRY — director, department of child and family welfare, Ministry of Social Affairs; head of elderly welfare, Cairo (ADVISOR)

FEDERAL REPUBLIC OF GERMANY

Prof. Erich LANG — head of medical clinic, Waldkrankenhaus St. Marien, Erlangen; president, German Gerontological Society (HEALTH)

Prof. Ursula LEHR — director, institute of psychology, University of Bonn; vice-president, German Gerontological Society (SOCIOLOGY)

Dr W. RUECKERT — head of socio-economic department, German Foundation for Care of the Aged, Köln (SOCIAL POLICY)

Prof. Hans THOMAE — director, institute of psychology, University of Bonn; president, International Association of Gerontology (ADVISOR)

FRANCE

Dr Françoise FORETTE — head, department of geriatrics, Hôpital Charles-Foix, Ivry; director, National Gerontology Foundation (HEALTH)

Prof. Michel PHILIBERT — professor of philosophy, University of Grenoble II (SOCIOLOGY)

Dr Pierre CHARBONNEAU — inspector-general of health; former director-general of health, Paris (SOCIAL POLICY)

Mlle Sophie VILLEMIN — multidisciplinary center of gerontology, Grenoble (ADVISOR)

INDIA

Dr J. D. PATHAK — director, medical research center, Bombay Hospital Trust, Bombay (HEALTH)

Prof. K. G. DESAI — head, department of personnel management and industrial relations, Tata Institute of Social Sciences, Bombay (SOCIOLOGY)

Prof. Ashok K. SAHNI — department of behavioral sciences and health management, Indian Institute of Management, Bangalore (SOCIAL POLICY)

ISRAEL

Prof. Michael DAVIES — director, Brookdale Institute; professor of medical ecology, Hebrew University, Jerusalem (HEALTH, COORDINATOR)

Ms Hannah WEIHL — researcher, Brookdale Institute; senior lecturer in social work (gerontology), Hebrew University, Jerusalem (SOCIOLOGY)

Prof. Shimon BERGMAN — professor of gerontology, University of Tel Aviv; director of education and training, Brookdale Institute (SOCIAL POLICY)

Mr Ya'akov KOP — researcher (social demography), Brookdale Institute (ADVISOR)

Additional advisors: — Dr Jean-Pierre BENDEL, Mr Haim FACTOR, Ms Patti SCHEIMER (rapporteur), Mr Amir SHMUELI, Ms Miriam SHTARKSHALL, Prof. Judith SHUVAL – Brookdale Institute; Dr M. SHADELL – American Joint Distribution Committee; Mr Yaron SOKOLOV – Israeli Association of Community Centers; Dr Samuel WARTSKI – Ministry of Health

ITALY

Prof. Gaetano CREPALDI — director, geriatric clinic, University of Padua (HEALTH)

Prof. Luigi AMADUCCI — director, neurology clinic, University of Florence; director "Aging brain" project national research center, Rome (SOCIOLOGY)

Prof. Renato LAZARRI — head, department of psychology, medical school, University of Rome (SOCIAL POLICY)

JAPAN

Prof. Mototaka MURAKAMI — director, Tokyo Metropolitan Geriatric Hospital (HEALTH)

Prof. Kazuo AOI — department of international and cultural studies, Tsuda College, Kodaira (SOCIOLOGY)

Dr Hideo IBE — director, Employees' Pension Fund Association, Tokyo (SOCIAL POLICY)

KENYA

Prof. Hilary P. OJIAMBO — head, department of cardiology, University of Nairobi (HEALTH)

Dr Walter ABILLA — senior lecturer, department of sociology, University of Nairobi (SOCIOLOGY)

The Hon. Dr Julia A. OJIAMBO, MP — assistant minister, Ministry of Housing and Social Services, Nairobi (SOCIAL POLICY)

NIGERIA

Dr Olatunji ADENIYI-JONES — health management consultant, Lagos; former director of health services, World Health Organization, Regional Office for Africa, Brazzaville (HEALTH, COORDINATOR)

Dr Olayiwola ERINOSHO — senior lecturer, department of sociology, University of Ibadan (SOCIOLOGY)

Mr David R. JACK — director of social development, Federal Ministry of Social Development, Youth, Sport, and Culture, Lagos (SOCIAL POLICY)

Dr Irene M. THOMAS — medical consultant, Lagos (ADVISOR)

Mr Benjamin OKAGBUE[†] — industrial consultant, Lagos (ADVISOR)

PHILIPPINES

Dr Rodolfo TALAG — member of board of directors, Philippine Association of Geriatrics and Gerontology, Manila (HEALTH)

Miss Adelina GO — assistant director, social research center, University of Santo Tomas, Manila (SOCIOLOGY)

Mrs Luvimin CUSTODIA — acting assistant director, bureau of rehabilitation, Ministry of Social Services and Development, Manila (SOCIAL POLICY)

† *deceased*

Mrs Sylvia MONTES — Minister of social services and development, Manila (ADVISOR)

POLAND

Prof. Halina SZWARC — director, institute of gerontology, main post-graduate medical center, Warsaw (HEALTH)

Dr Joanna STAREGA-PIASEK — department of sociology, University of Warsaw (SOCIOLOGY)

Prof. Wojciech PENDICH — head, department of gerontology, medical school, Bialystok (SOCIAL POLICY)

Prof. Zbigniew BRZEZINSKI — department of epidemiology and public health, National Institute of Hygiene, Warsaw (COORDINATOR)

Prof. Jan KOSTRZEWSKI — department of epidemiology, National Institute of Hygiene; secretary, medical division, Polish Academy of Sciences, Warsaw (ADVISOR)

SWEDEN

Prof. Alvar SVANBORG — department of geriatric medicine, University of Göteborg (HEALTH)

Dr Dam MALSTROEM — department of geriatric medicine and long-term care, Vasa Hospital, Göteborg (SOCIOLOGY)

Mr Douglas SKALIN — head of section, Swedish Planning and Rationalization Institute of the Health and Social Services, Stockholm (SOCIAL POLICY)

UK

Prof. John GRIMLEY EVANS — department of medicine and geriatrics, General Hospital, Newcastle-upon-Tyne (HEALTH)

Prof. Margot JEFFERYS — director, social research unit, Bedford College, London (SOCIOLOGY)

Dr Eric MIDWINTER — secretary, Centre for Policy on Aging, London (SOCIAL POLICY)

Dr Tony J. SMITH — deputy editor, British Medical Journal, London (MODERATOR and RAPPORTEUR)

EXPERTS

USA

Prof. Robert KANE — department of medicine and public health, University of California, Los Angeles; senior researcher, Rand Corporation, Santa Monica, California (HEALTH)

Prof. George MADDOX — director, Center for the Study of Aging and Human Development, Duke University Medical Center, Durham, North Carolina (SOCIOLOGY)

Prof. Robert BINSTOCK — director, Policy Center on Aging; Stulberg professor of law and politics, Brandeis University, Waltham, Massachusetts (SOCIAL POLICY)

Biographies

Philip Selby is a British physician and a former scientific writer and editor with the World Health Organization, Geneva. He is responsible for community medicine and epidemiology with the Sandoz Institute.

Mal Schechter is an American journalist who has contributed to lay and professional journals on health and socio-economic affairs in the field of aging, and is an expert consultant with the National Institute on Aging, Washington, D.C. He has just been appointed to help lead an aging-policy institute within the new department of geriatrics and adult development, at Mount Sinai school of medicine, New York.

Jean-Jacques Vollbrecht is a Swiss economist and business administrator and is project manager with Sandoz Ltd. He is temporarily attached to the Sandoz Institute.

Raymond Rigoni is a Swiss lawyer specializing in pharmaceutical legislation. He is director of the Sandoz Institute and head of external relations for the pharmaceutical division of Sandoz Ltd.

Adrian Griffiths is a British economist and a former lecturer at the London School of Hygiene and Tropical Medicine. He is responsible for health management and economics with the Sandoz Institute.